LONERS, LOSERS, AND LOVERS

Elderly Tenants in a Slum Hotel

JOYCE STEPHENS

Loners, Losers, and Lovers

ELDERLY TENANTS IN A SLUM HOTEL

UNIVERSITY OF WASHINGTON PRESS
SEATTLE AND LONDON

This book was published with the assistance of a grant from the Andrew
W. Mellon Foundation.

Library of Congress Cataloging in Publication Data

Stephens, Joyce, 1941-
    Loners, losers, and lovers.

    Bibliography: p.
    1. Aged—United States—Case studies. 2. Aged—United States—Dwel-
lings—Case studies. 3. Aged—Psychology—Case studies. 4. Old age
homes—United States. I. Title.
HQ1064.U5S73   301.43'5   75-40874
ISBN 0-295-95494-9

TO HEMINGWAY AND HELEN,
WITH GRATITUDE AND RESPECT

They city sidewalkers
straight striding unglancers
feral thoughted afternooners
(every
each run a one box
for only lonelitude)

"Lebensraum"
Robert Stephens, 1972

Foreword

A sociologist who reads a manuscript written by another sociologist for an audience that extends beyond the discipline approaches it with both high hope and deep skepticism. We would like to be able to communicate insights from our perspective beyond our midst, but usually we fail. The failure can often be attributed to an obsession with abstract concepts that leads to a masking of the social experience that we are attempting to comprehend. Concepts thus become an end in themselves rather than a tool to unlock understanding.

Joyce Stephens has overcome all my natural skepticism. She has succeeded where others have failed. *Loners, Losers, and Lovers* is a remarkable sociological book. For once, sociological concepts and methods have been used in an unobtrusive way to probe into and capture the essence of an obscure but important social phenomenon. Even sociologists who do not subscribe to the "symbolic interactionist" approach will, I believe, recognize and applaud a masterful demonstration of how this framework yields understandings and insights not garnered by other methods.

This book is a contribution to knowledge; but it is more than that. It is a luminous, lucid human document containing startling sketches of high drama in low places. Aging is something we all, sooner or later, must come to terms with. This book, while dealing with a very special population, addresses general issues in a profound way.

Take, for example, the findings of this study that post a major challenge to the traditional conception of the "aging process," one that emphasizes the return to dependency and passivity said to be characteristic of the elderly. That conception is derived from studies of the *institutionalized aged* who, in the author's terms, *"are* passive, terrified, and dependent, and they do slip away irrevocably from the world of the living." How is it, then, that the elderly denizens of the deteriorating inner core of our cities, sitting in their lonely rooms in run-down hotels, manage to defy this process despite an environment that bristles with hostility and is marked by alienation and anonymity? Or, briefly put, how can they be both "losers" and "survivors"?

The answers, which will no doubt surprise many readers, arise from sensitive, systematic, clearly articulated observations that reveal in fascinating detail remarkable capacities for developing a variety of successful coping strategies. "Participant observation" succeeds in doing this because the investigator manages with skill to mine the meanings of the participants of this "world of the alone" in their terms, terms that illuminate and indict conventional institutional arrangements and inform us not only about the problems of the aged but also provide new insights into urban structure, collective processes, role theory, sex differentiation, and social deviance.

In the end, however, it is the life-style of the aged occupants of the old hotels that leaves the large impression. Embedded as they are in a fierce environment peopled by petty thieves, pimps, prostitutes, addicts, and hustlers, their privacy and independence yields a toughness and dignity that add up to survival. It does not detract from this study to question to what degree the genesis of these traits preceeded or followed the entry of the aged into this environment.

Other haunting questions remain. Is survival enough? While this life-style sustains self, what does that mean for society?

Every reader of this book will be forced to reflect on the implications of this study. If conventional institutions are deficient, surely it cannot be said that the arrangements portrayed here are sufficient. Left to themselves, these aged do cope and their character commands respect. But is this the best that a society can do in response to the growing numbers and the growing problems of the aged?

OTTO N. LARSEN
Department of Sociology
University of Washington

Preface

Social scientists have become increasingly cognizant of the failure of institutions to meet the needs of people. Concomitant with this growing awareness of the inadequacies of our institutions, there has been developing a voluminous body of knowledge explicating the general dimensions and specific characteristics of those groups in America who most suffer from the inadequacies of institutional arrangements.

Of the groups whose unmet needs bombard us with painful regularity, the aged American is one of the most prominent. The old represent the obsolete, the cast off and cast out. The old inherit the full consequences of a society whose institutions serve not human needs, but rather technological demands. In a society that routinely renders human resources and skills obsolete, the aged possess abilities that come to be defined as no longer contributory. The institutionalization of this cultural obsolescence has profound and far-reaching implications for the status of the old, in that they are perceived as expendable in a society geared toward "progress," innovation, and change. These devaluing societal definitions, in turn, become internalized in the self-definitions of the old.

Social scientists have only recently turned their interest to the condition of the aged American. Prior to the 1950s, few research efforts were directed toward understanding the problems confronting the elderly. However, along with the upsurge in research interest in the sociological correlates of minorities in American society, there has been a growing concern with identifying and analyzing the characteristics of the aged minority. Further contributing to this current research interest has been the phenomenal increase in the number of older persons in our society. The average life expectancy of Americans has increased by twenty-one years since 1900. In 1900 there were approximately three million (4.1 percent of the total population) Americans who were sixty-five or older. In 1970 this number had increased to twenty million (10 percent of the population), which was the fastest rate of increase of any age category except children between the ages of five and fourteen.

The situation of many elderly Americans is bleak in the extreme. They are poor, undereducated, and living in substandard housing. The rapidity of industrial and technological change has produced a "lost generation" of the old. In the years since they occupied the positions of power and made the decisions, the dimensions of our society have changed in major ways. "Progress" has rendered obsolete the technical skills they mastered.* Our older citizens find themselves excluded from productive work, and they suffer the inevitable devaluation which follows.

Our society is faced with the complex task of reintegrating into the mainstream of American life large numbers of men and women, already aged, who can anticipate another full decade of life. Industrial society has created a new social group, but the culture that gave birth to this group has yet to find ways of incorporating it into the ongoing social system. The aged constitute a significant group in our society; their problems present an important challenge to social scientists committed to the advancement of a society in which people are able to meet their

---

* For a particularly vivid portrait of the consequences of growing old in America, the reader is urged to read the final section of Henry, *Culture Against Man*. His position that the status of the old is the expectable outcome of pathologies of a cultural nature is well argued.

needs and live fully human lives.

Despite the increasing interest of social scientists and the growing volume of literature on the aged, one category of elderly Americans has been overlooked, namely, those who live in old, deteriorating hotels in large urban centers. Yet there is evidence that an increasing number of the aged are choosing converted hotels as their place of residence.

Old, once prosperous hotels that have become the victims of competition from motels and suburban hotels, have in many cities been unable to survive by catering to a transient clientele. Consequently, they have had to accept a clientele that is more or less permanent in character. A large proportion of these "permanent guests" are in the ranks of the elderly. Given that these converted hotels generally provide the lowest rates that unaided private enterprise has yet been able to furnish, it is to be expected that they will continue to house a growing number of the urban aged.

Typically these single-room-occupancy slum hotels (SROs) are located in the central city in deteriorating neighborhoods with high crime rates and low income rates. SROs provide little in the way of either medical or recreational services to their aged tenants. However, they do provide shelter and a certain privacy and autonomy for the aged urban poor.

Little is known of the sociological characteristics of these hotels, and even less of their occupants. This group of the elderly, therefore, represents a source of potential research interest. Since the group does constitute a growing segment of the elderly, and, in addition, one that has received almost no study at all, I concluded that a study of the relevant sociological correlates of the SRO hotel would constitute a valuable and important research project. To this end, I investigated the social world of the elderly tenants of an SRO situated in a large midwestern city. Interactional patterns were identified and then analyzed for their meanings in an effort to determine the part they play in the aged person's repertoire of coping strategies and skills. Of particular interest to me were the available roles within the SRO society, the stability of role patterns, supporting norms and values that serve to maintain relationships and control deviance, the importance of coping mechanisms, isolation, and the nature of the relationships between the tenants and the "outside." Thus, the scope of my research sought to include all of the social arrangements that the aged SRO tenants developed to generate and sustain roles and relational activities, and to cope with personal problems associated with the aging process.

The realization of the goal of this study—a descriptive analysis of the social world of the aged SRO tenant—may act as a catalyst for other social scientists interested in the sociology of the aging. Certainly, it is both my intention and my hope that this exploration into the "world of the alone" will be a pioneering journey that both contributes to and, equally important, encourages further research into this neglected area.

Acknowledgments

I am indebted to the elderly tenants of the Guinevere, whose book this is. That their story is to be told at all was made possible by their willingness to participate. If I have been faithful in the telling, then some small measure of repayment may be made.

In particular, I wish to thank my principal informants, whose patience and insight corrected false steps. I am grateful to the manager of the Guinevere whose valuable (if cynical) cooperation aided in the gathering of preliminary material.

Dr. Frank Hartung and Dr. Leon Warshay aided me greatly by their much-appreciated noninterference in the research. Their willingness to allow freedom and latitude in the development of the study underscored the confidence they had in the worth of the research.

I wish to thank Wally Smith for providing a richly humanistic atmosphere that was supportive of my work.

Dave Hartman aided me by providing a tape recorder and by triggering ideas that were to add provocatively to the study.

Early versions of several chapters appeared in the following journals, whose permission to reprint I gratefully acknowledge: "On Being Excluded: An Analysis of Elderly and Adolescent Street Hustlers" (with Clifford English), *Urban Life and Culture*, vol. 4, no. 2 (July 1975); "Romance in the SRO," *The*

ACKNOWLEDGMENTS

Gerontologist, vol. 14, no. 4; "Making It in the SRO: Survival Strategies of Elderly Tenants of a Slum Hotel," *Australian and New Zealand Journal of Sociology,* vol. 10, no. 3; "Society of the Alone: Privacy, Freedom, and Utilitarianism as Dominant Norms in the SRO," *Journal of Gerontology;* "Carnies and Marks: The Sociology of Elderly Street Peddlers," *Sociological Symposium,* Spring 1974.

To Rob, I can only say that you, most of all, understood the meaning of this book and why it was written. You have suffered its birth, and you have rejoiced in its maturation.

Contents

LONERS, LOSERS, AND LOVERS
Elderly Tenants in a Slum Hotel

CHAPTER ONE

"One of Your Better Low-Class Hotels"

When I moved into the Guinevere Hotel,[1] the tenants, with an irony that is typical, informed me that it was "one of your better low-class hotels." The Guinevere is a deteriorating single-room-occupancy hotel situated in the inner core of a large midwestern American city. Over a half-century old, the Guinevere reached its apogee in the 1920s, when it was considered to be one of the better hotels in the city, and catered to a wealthy if notorious clientele. Hoodlums, gangsters, and the like, "Legs" Diamond and members of the Purple Gang, were frequent guests at the hotel and earned it a certain notoriety.

With the decline of this turbulent era, the Guinevere fell upon lean times and began to deteriorate. During the forties and fifties, it was given the nickname of the "riding stable," as it became well-known in the area as a hotel catering to seekers of illicit sexual services. In addition, a physician operated a profitable abortion ring out of the hotel until he was convicted.

The present owners maintain a number of hotels in the city. They have attempted to arrest the rapidly degenerating operation of the Guinevere and to quell the scandal produced by the violent death of its previous owner, who was beaten to death in her room. They have been able to keep the Guinevere afloat

1. All names and references to places have been fictionalized to insure the anonymity of individuals.

by catering to a growing number of permanent, elderly occupants, so that at present less than two-thirds of the tenants are transients.

The surrounding neighborhood is honeycombed with rooming houses and hotels catering to transients, blacks, alcoholics, addicts, hustlers, prostitutes, recently migrated southern families, and the elderly poor. The economic character of the area is revealed in the high concentration of marginal businesses—nudie shows, nude photographic studios, resale shops, cheap cafes and restaurants, dry-cleaning stores, "we buy anything" shops, and bars. The area contains a heavy concentration of social and psychological pathology. Addicts and winos can be seen nodding off in alleys and in the backs of vandalized cars on the side streets. Street crime is common, even routine: muggings and robberies, frequently involving severe beatings and even killings, are a constant source of anxiety to the residents. Street brawls are a daily occurrence. Fires are so common in the cheap hotels and rooming houses that they scarcely stir the resident's interest. The bombing of a cafe adjacent to the Guinevere evoked minor expressions of regret that the cheapest cup of coffee in the neighborhood was now gone. The ubiquitous violence and the myriad forms of social and personal deviance have a direct effect on the attitudes and life styles of the people and give to the area an atmosphere of mutual suspicion and fear.

The Guinevere has eleven floors, with a total of 524 rooms. During my research, 371 rooms were occupied, of which 108 were rented to aged tenants. There are two wings, separated by two interconnected lobbies. Both lobbies have outside doors, but one is locked every evening at six o'clock. Anyone entering or leaving at night must use one door, which is in full view of the reception desk. Each wing is serviced by two self-service elevators that are inclined to frequent breakdowns.

In addition to the two lobbies, the Guinevere has a bar, a dry-cleaning service, a television room, a small room in one lobby out of which a bookie operates, and a restaurant that is physically connected to the hotel but is operated independently. In the lobbies are several vending machines that dispense coffee, cigarettes, candy bars, and soft drinks.

Rents are comparable to other hotels in the neighborhood ranging from sixteen dollars a week for a sleeping room to forty-six dollars a week for a two-bedroom suite. The expensive (by comparison) suites are usually vacant. Rooms fall into four categories: (1) sleeping rooms, which have no bath facilities, provide once-a-week maid service, and range in price from sixteen dollars weekly without television to eighteen dollars with black-and-white television to twenty dollars with color television; (2) connectors, which share a bath, provide once-a-week maid service, and range in price from twenty dollars weekly without television to twenty-two dollars with black-and-white television to twenty-four dollars with color television; (3) private rooms, which have a bath, daily maid service, and range in price from twenty-four dollars weekly without television to twenty-six dollars with black-and-white television to twenty-eight dollars with color television; and (4) suites, which have a bath, daily maid service, color television, and rent for forty dollars weekly for one bedroom and forty-six dollars for two bedrooms. The majority of the 108 elderly permanents live in the cheapest rooms and pay an average rent of $20.59 a week. Most live in sleeping rooms, although some live in connectors and a few have private rooms.

There are two public bathrooms (shower and commode) on each floor, one for men and one for women. However, more often than not the tenants disregard this sexual division of the communal bathrooms. This may not seem surprising in view of the sex ratio of ninety-seven males to eleven females. The units have neither cooking facilities nor refrigerators. All rooms contain a bed, a wash basin, a dresser, and a chair. The furniture is cheap and generally in need of repair. Paint is peeling off the walls, and cockroaches are abundant. During the winter months, rooms above the fourth floor are inadequately heated. The halls are dimly lit, and robberies and fights in these dark stretches are not uncommon. All doors have double locks.

The aged tenants are scattered throughout the hotel, although the manager attempts to put those with more severe disabilities (poor vision, paralysis) on the bottom four floors. In general, the hotel maintains a policy of not renting to elderly who are not ambulatory, although exceptions are made. The seventh floor is informally reserved for what the manager describes as his "nuts and mentals." There are four black tenants. The area has a high concentration of blacks, but the manager resolutely refuses to rent to them because "They're troublemakers and they frighten my old people."

The average age is sixty-seven, and the oldest resident is ninety-one. The length of residence ranges from two to fifty-one years, with a mean of nine years. A significant proportion of the elderly tenants moved to the Guinevere from nearby hotels, and, indeed, this pattern of shuffling from one hotel to another is fairly common in the area. Among the males, over half have never been married, and the remainder are divorced or widowed. The females include a larger proportion of widowed or divorced.

Health problems are endemic in this group. The major core of diseases includes the geriatric illnesses (arteriosclerotic disease, stroke, and rheumatoid disorders), sensory deficits (poor vision, auditory loss), alcoholism, and various forms and degrees of paralysis. In addition, a significant minority suffers from mental illness, including schizophrenia, paranoid disorders, and the depressive syndromes. Many of them are in need of prosthetic devices (glasses, hearing aids, canes, dental appliances), but have neither the income nor the personal resources to obtain them.

Their work histories are generally episodic and encompass a variety of marginal work situations. Few had occupational careers in a formal sense: for the most part, they were concentrated in low-paying, intermittent types of employment—vendors, carnival hustlers, spot laborers, seasonal workers, petty criminals. For most, retirement was not an event that occurred on a particular day and terminated a career; rather, it happened gradually as they became less and less able to find even low-paying jobs, including street vending, spot labor, "go-fors," and the many forms of hustling. Over 80 percent are on some form of state assistance. Their income is low, with the major sources being Old Age Assistance (OAA), social security, disability insurance, and money picked up from occasional jobs. A small portion receive pensions.

Despite the prevalence of medical and psychiatric disabilities and the low economic status, a comparison of this group with other aged SRO tenants in the area would reveal that, as a group, they are not the most severely disadvantaged. The Union Hotel and the Lock Hotel, both adjacent to the Guinevere, house many former Guinevere residents. Tenants who become a problem to the management because of their accelerating alcoholic bouts, repeated failures to pay rent, or constant public brawling with other tenants, are eventually put out. Most likely they will seek lodging in one of these neighboring hotels. Thus, despite the comparable economic status of tenants, these nearby hotels contain many Guinevere rejects. As the manager and the tenants say, the Guinevere is "one of your better low-class hotels" in the area.

The attitudes of the elderly tenants toward the Guinevere betray a curious mixture of grudging appreciation and discomfiture. They are involved in a kind of love-hate relationship with the hotel and its functionaries. On the one hand, they view the "Rock" as their personal turf where no one will bother them and they can live their lives in privacy and autonomy; on the other hand, they are aware of the justifiably questionable reputation of this slum hotel. They are aware of the low repute in which such hotels, and by association their occupants, are held; however, they rationalize this stigmatizing attitude by pointing out that people from the "outside" cannot possibly understand or know what it is like in the hotel and that outsiders are guilty of accepting erroneous myths about the character of both the hotel and its residents. This strong ambivalence pervades their feelings about the hotel.

Undoubtedly, one of the major advantages of hotel living for these people lies in the autonomy that is characteristic of hotels —they are free to determine their own schedules; they may eat when they want, come and go as they will, without interference from anyone. Their only supervision is themselves, and they enjoy the continued opportunity to make their own decisions. In the words of one seventy-two-year-old woman who has lived in the Guinevere more than fourteen years: "One good thing about living here is you can live your own private life, and no one will bother you. You can be more private than if you lived in your own home. Outsiders think a lot of mistaken ideas about people in hotels. They can't know, they are wrong in those . . . er . . . opinions about the people in hotels. These are *our* homes, we live *here*."

Hotel life encourages personal freedom and privacy; in addition, it frees the tenants from certain tasks that are necessary in other private living arrangements, such as minimal housework. A sixty-eight-year-old man on OAA who has been at the Guinevere for six years put it this way: "Everything is right here. If I lived in the suburbs, what would I do, how would I get around?" A former carnival vendor had this to say: "I could live free in a house my niece has but I'll stay here, where things are cookin'. I'm independent. Some old people just give up, but I'm always plottin' and plannin' . . . and the 'Rock' has elevators. You don't have to walk up stairs." An elderly cabdriver who had moved out of the Guinevere, taken an apartment, and then later moved back into the hotel, gave his reasons for preferring to live in a hotel: "It was too quiet in my apartment, and too much work, washing and cooking and such. But, I missed the people here and the comings and goings."

There is an element of living there to "be with your own kind," which is sometimes expressed in the movement from another hotel to the Guinevere. A commonly held belief is that families and children do not really want to be bothered with the old people. Suburbs are for the young and for families; the old feel awkward there. In the anonymity of an inner-city slum hotel, absolute privacy and a high degree of personal freedom can be relished.

Further, the hotel situation provides access to services which the elderly tenants believe would constitute a problem in different living situations—transportation, proximity to the downtown area, maid service, company when desired and privacy when preferred, freedom, a certain anonymity, their "own kind," and "happenings." Many of these elderly people have been unable to live peacefully with their families, and the greater latitude permitted in the impersonal atmosphere of the hotel is an important factor in their continued residence. There they may act out behaviors that family members would have resisted, for example, excessive drinking, consorting with prostitutes, and other less extravagant behaviors which have been deemed as inappropriate for the old in our age-myopic society. In addition, for a number of them, relative isolation and unwillingness to enter into social commitments have been lifelong patterns.

Many elderly tenants express the attitude that the Guinevere is going to be the final period of their lives. They do not anticipate or plan on leaving:

> The Guinevere is the road of no return. Old-timers come to this point of their life. This is the last place they'll ever stay. When they get here, they don't never leave.
>
> A lot of us come down here to do this or that with the intention of leaving, but we keep coming back and at last, we never leave.
>
> This is a place where people come to die.

Generally, they view the Guinevere as "nicer" than other hotels in the area, pointing out that in the Guinevere people do not "jungle up." ("Jungling up" refers to the practice of communal cooking and eating of meals among hotel occupants, which occurs in some of the SRO hotels that cater to the most

9

indigent groups of alcoholic elderly. The practice is virtually nonexistent in the Guinevere.) However, there are dissenting opinions on this matter, especially among the tenants who have lived at the Guinevere longer than a decade. They feel that the hotel has deteriorated, pointing out that undesirables are no longer screened out, that "they let anybody and everybody in, even prostitutes." They complain that the hotel's standards have gone down, and that many people who live there would have been turned away earlier. There is general agreement among all of the tenants that the neighborhood is deteriorating, and that inevitably the hotel will go downhill.

The manager acknowledges this loss of selectivity in clientele by noting that it was financially necessary to liberalize the policy regarding who would be allowed in, and that this has resulted in a gradual change in the type of people living there. This includes the acceptance of what the manager identifies as "welfare types," homosexuals, prostitutes, and drunks. The manager's formal policy is that prostitutes may live in the hotel as long as they do not ply their trade inside the hotel. In actual practice, the manager, like most managers of slum hotels, ignores prostitution unless it begins to encroach upon his business operation. Thus, when complaints become numerous or several tenants are unable to pay their rent, he checks, and if he finds that a prostitute in the hotel has been getting his rent money, he "cleans them out" of the hotel. In general, though, the Guinevere management is liberal and tolerant in its treatment of "hookers." Indeed, one of the tenants' more colorful nicknames for the Guinevere is the "whortel."

Specific dissatisfactions with the hotel include complaints about the inadequacy of heat in winter, noisy tenants, people throwing trash and debris from the windows, cockroaches, and fights in the elevators or halls. Some of the tenants feel that the current management has arrested the hotel's decline. They speak of the manager with grudging approval, for they see several changes that he has made which they interpret as efforts to provide services for them. Examples include vending machines in the lobbies, free ice to residents, and the inauguration of a Saturday raffle, at which time a tenant wins two free tickets to a current sports event and a five-dollar bill. This has generated a modest enthusiasm among some of the men. Another change effected by the manager was his handling of the hotel "hermits." These elderly tenants, many bedridden, never left their rooms and paid maids to bring them food. According to several sources, their fingernails grew to great lengths. The current manager had them moved into hospitals and nursing homes.

If there is ambivalence in their assessment of the relative advantages and disadvantages of living in the hotel, the tenants are unanimous in their evaluation that at least the Guinevere is a better place to live than the other hotels in the area, and that any hotel, however dilapidated, is superior to any nursing home. The common assertion is that the tenants at the Guinevere are a "better class of people" and that other nearby hotels are *really* "low-class." Since several of them have lived in these other hotels, they know from experience the relatively better treatment and services provided at the Guinevere. The Guinevere is cleaner, repairs are made sooner, there are fewer building code violations, and all rooms are equipped with telephones, yet the rent is comparable. The manager's attitude toward these people appears nearly benevolent when contrasted with that of some other SRO managers. The following excerpt from an interview with the manager of an adjacent hotel is revealing: "These old people! Who'd be interested in them? These old people are poor: they've always been poor; they elected it; they prefer it. They've never contributed to society. They're single, never even raised a family; they aren't even has-beens, they never were. They don't eat right; they never ate right. They've never been anywhere, never done anything. All they've done is take up space. I've contributed. At least, I've paid a lot of taxes."

The tenants are unanimously hostile and suspicious toward nursing homes. To these fiercely independent people, nursing homes represent the loss of autonomy they are determined to avoid. They frequently contrast their own independent living arrangements with their ideas of what nursing homes are like. Their basic view is that nursing homes exploit old people. A sentiment commonly expresses is that the time is approaching when old people will lose their independence, and the government will foist upon them programs that will serve not their interests but rather political aims. Nursing homes are the prime example, as far as they are concerned. The tenants regularly draw comparisons between the Guinevere and the two nursing homes in the immediate area. They call these homes "playpens" where "they tell you when to get up, when to eat, where to go, and take your money." By contrast, several Guinevere permanents characterized themselves as "lone wolves," "independent loners," and variations of this idea.

For these people, nursing homes also represent the tangible expression of society's rejection of old people. The following are representative comments of tenants on the subject:

> They are the final humiliation for old people, the final humiliation.

> Oh, the playpens, where people tell you when to get up, when to breathe. They take your money, yeah, I sold a rubber [balloon] to a woman lives at the Shady Glen, and they came out and said they'd arrest me if I came around again. Said she wasn't right and I took advantage of her. Ha, they said I couldn't take her money, couldn't sell her that rubber, but they take all her money.

> Old people are not wanted. Nobody wants us old geezers. So, they, ah, segregate us, in nursing homes or ghettos. Oh, and the homes are terrible places where they tell you what to do. And what you want doesn't matter at all.

The specter of institutionalization looms as a reminder of the catastrophic consequences of loss of personal determination. It is an admission of dependency and physical and mental failure.

Interestingly, they make little mention of specific disadvantages or conditions (poor food, abuse, and so forth). In fact, few have actually lived in such places—although most know people who do. Rather, they object in principle to the very idea of homes for the aged, with their characteristic programs of regimented activities. Some distrust of social service agencies is generated by the issue of nursing home placement; some of the tenants fear that social workers will push them into a home. To quote a seventy-three-year-old retired cabdriver who has lived in the Guinevere since 1964: "Social workers would likely tell us this hotel is a bad environ [*sic*] for us, and we don't like it that they're always questioning our competences [*sic*], and saying this is a bad place, and we'd be better off in one of them homes."

The distrust and in some cases hostility of these elderly toward social workers was communicated to me in the early days of field work. Many of the tenants assumed that I was a social worker (an improvement perhaps on their initial belief that I was a hooker) and were consequently aloof and inaccessible. Fortunately, their suspicions relaxed as they observed my behavior, and later one elderly individual summed up their assessment of my presence there: "Oh well, that's all right. You're no social worker. Writin' a book that's O.K. You aren't going to hurt us."

CHAPTER TWO

The Man in the Seersucker Suit

With the exception of a brief flurry of interest that emerged prior to World Wars I and II and then subsided, there have been few attempts to study SRO society. Arnold M. Rose noted the lack of interest in the problems of the urban unattached, a segment of our population that is overrepresented in SROs.[1] His brief historical review of the disinterest shown toward this group demonstrates the difficulties experienced by researchers concerned with this area. We know little of the life styles and social system of this population. Rose identified the obvious characteristics of such slum hotels: the rent is relatively cheap; the furniture is cheap and sparse; sanitary facilities are often outmoded and insufficient; vermin are prevalent; and rooms vary greatly in cleanliness. Of the life styles and concerns of the tenants, Rose has little to say, other than to note that their lives are spent in privacy, social isolation, and anonymity.

Norman S. Hayner, in a rather fanciful book on hotel living, pointed out the atomistic character of hotel society.[2] He noted that the lack of social solidarity among the tenants of urban hotels leads to a kind of "moral holiday" in which individual goals and interests are pursued at the expense of communal

1. Rose, "Interest in the Living Arrangements of the Urban Unattached"; Rose, "Living Arrangements of Unattached Persons."
2. Hayner, *Hotel Life*.

goals. Concomitant with the loosening of "the moral binding force of consensual norms" is the high frequency of "acting out" behaviors, often bordering on the illegal. Hayner also stressed the social isolation, impersonality, and anonymity of the world of the hotel tenant.

Harvey W. Zorbaugh designated the "dweller in furnished rooms" as a social type.[3] He characterized the world of this group as socially impoverished and colored by an extreme degree of isolation, anonymity, and mutual distrust. Zorbaugh's analysis included the tenants of hotels and rooming houses, and was not geared specifically to the aged tenants of SROs.

Two studies of SROs in New York City by Joan Shapiro cast more light on the specific characteristics of the aged SRO tenant.[4] Shapiro described this group as characterized by social and psychological maladaptation and chronic physical disease. An overwhelming percentage were receiving welfare payments. A large proportion (over 50 percent) were alcoholics. Hunger was pervasive among them. The ever-present violence contributed to their mutual fear and distrust. With regard to social groupings, Shapiro identified common pathology as the basis of association; three groups emerged—winos, addicts, and "mentals." A recurrent pattern was the clustering of a group of alcoholic males around an older nonalcoholic female, who both mothered and disciplined them. Around such strong females, quasi "families" developed, offering a modicum of protection, affection, and economic sustenance to the members. Shapiro summarized the life style of these SRO occupants as one of passive watchfulness that barely masked fear, resentment, and suspicion.

The overall portrait of SRO dwellers that emerges from these earlier studies is one of individuals who live in a society marked by extreme degrees of isolation and impersonality. With regard to these characteristics, the Guinevere tenants are

3. Zorbaugh, "The Dweller in Furnished Rooms."
4. Shapiro, "Single-room Occupancy"; Shapiro, "Dominant Leaders Among Slum Hotel Residents."

representative of other SRO populations. The interpersonal world of the elderly tenants of the Guinevere includes the dominant features of freedom, utilitarianism, and isolation. They maintain relationships which are markedly instrumental in nature; and, as will become apparent, the emphasis upon utilitarian, nonintimate social ties is an essential tool in a highly developed strategy of survival. With few exceptions, there is little group cohesiveness or solidarity binding the tenants of the Guinevere together. This pattern of relative isolation and fragmentation reflects the specific exigencies of hotel society.

There are two significant groups with whom the SRO tenant must deal on a day-to-day basis, and with whom reciprocal expectations and norms must be worked out. The first group includes those people connected with the operation of the hotel—the manager and the staff people, such as desk clerks, porters, maintenance people, switchboard operators, and bartenders. The other SRO tenants form the second group, which includes both transients and permanent "guests" in the Guinevere or neighboring SRO hotels. These two groups are the people who compose the core of the hotel society, and it is in relationship to them that mutual roles and norms are worked out to form the network of interpersonal ties. Additionally, there are peripheral types, such as social workers, police officers, prostitutes, and owners of nearby cafes and bars.

The finding that the relationships of these elderly are instrumental in nature is understandable in the face of the constant need to mobilize extremely limited resources to maintain minimal living conditions in an antagonistic environment.[5] Social bonds are relatively impoverished, and their primary function is the attainment of goods and services. These relationships are, then, fundamentally economic, in the broad sense. Any consideration of the relational bonds formed in this hotel society must recognize these facts.

The world of the SRO tenant is basically atomistic; the

5. Chapter 3 deals at length with the issue of maintenance of self in the hostile environment of the SRO hotel.

fabric of social relationships is thin and fragile. The lack of group cohesiveness creates a world of strangers acting in terms of their individual interests, rather than pairs or larger groupings acting for shared goals.

The form of interaction between the aged tenants in the Guinevere and the management is prototypical of other relationships: it is instrumental and atomistic. The tenant's goal is to cultivate favor in order to get something, and this is best accomplished by forming individual relationships. Despite the presence of official hotel policies—such as paying the rent on time and one week in advance, not allowing prostitutes in the hotel, the forbidding of spitting in the public areas of the hotel, and the like—the actual enforcement of hotel rules varies greatly. The cultivation of management's favor can result in the bending of these rules. The atomistic quality of this system is especially apparent in those situations where there are common grievances; tenants in no way act collectively, rather they attempt individually to ameliorate these aggravations for themselves. The social structure at the Guinevere is not penetrable by groups with grievance lists, but it is receptive to individuals —individuals who have in a pragmatic and deliberate fashion nurtured management's benevolence.

Because the hotel management plays such a significant part in the survival measures of these aged poor, the nature of the social ties is symptomatic of the overall individualistic and pragmatic framework of relationships. These tenants take care of their needs and survive strictly as individuals, not as a result of cooperative and organized action. Gerontologists have long noted the disinclination of the elderly to join groups, their tendency to renounce relationships, their indifference to collective action in their behalf. Typically, the explanations for these prominent patterns are variations of the "inherent consequences of the aging process" theme. Yet, as we understand more clearly the totality of situational features that surround and confront the aging individual, we recognize the inadequacy of such explanations. In the society of the Guinevere, the disinclination of the aged tenants to act as a group to get what they want cannot be explained by the presumed alienating effects of an aging process. Rather, it is an adjustment to a social structure that would be unreceptive to such tactics.

The key figure representing management in the Guinevere is the hotel manager, Mr. Christmas, not so fondly nicknamed by his tenants, "the man in the seersucker suit." All exchanges between the tenants and the hotel management are in his jurisdiction; he is the one authority with whom the tenants have to contend. Mr. Christmas attempts to know everything that is going on in the hotel, and he does not hesitate to use his knowledge to bully tenants into doing what he wants. One technique he uses is public ridicule, usually in the hotel lobby, where a good-sized audience may gather to hear him loudly and profanely upbraid a tenant for some violation of hotel rules.

The manager's control over the operation of the hotel is aided by the willingness of various staff members and tenants to act as spies. Referred to as "bird dogs" by other tenants, these individuals report to the manager the happenings that will interest him. Their reportage is sporadic and is often precipitated either by an attempt to get even with another tenant for some real or imagined wrong, or by an attempt to identify with management and thus to demonstrate superiority over the other tenants. The rewards for such espionage are thus vengeance or the proclamation of status differences. Two illustrative examples of this are Mrs. Macken and Mr. Nice. Mrs. Macken, the oldest resident of the Guinevere, who is from a wealthy family, displays open contempt for the other tenants, and makes it clear that she, at any rate, does not belong to this class of people. Mr. Nice reports on anyone with whom he happens to be at odds. The tenants' opinions of these spies shift from resentment to half-hearted pity for the "poor old things." From the viewpoint of management, they are frequently more annoying than they are reliable or informative; nevertheless, no particular effort is made to discourage them.

While the manager is determined to know everything that

goes on in his hotel, the tenants, for the most part, try to have as little to do with him as possible, at least until they desire some favor from him, in which case they will usually approach him directly. The basis for relationships between the manager and the tenants resides in the usefulness of each to the other. The manager wants tenants who pay on time, do not cause trouble, do not break the furniture, do not bring the police, do not upset other tenants; and he wants a full house. The tenants, in turn, expect protection, privacy, freedom, and a minimal degree of comfort. They are dependent upon each other to realize these goals.

Accompanying the behavior of manager and tenant with respect to one another are other-defining attitudes which buttress the fundamentally wary stance of relationships. Thus, the manager, while acknowledging certain differences in renting to an elderly clientele, defines both his old permanents and his younger transients as belonging in the same social category. For him, the tenants in his hotel constitute a social "type." They are losers and misfits, people who have in seriously damaging ways failed to fit into the norms of the larger society. The manager frequently pointed out to me young people in the hotel who "are going to spend the rest of their lives here." In his view, there are basically three groups living in the Guinevere—"welfare bums," "veteran bums," and "old bums." He attributes the pronounced reluctance of many of his tenants to reveal their backgrounds to their having been either in prisons or in asylums. With regard to the old tenants, Mr. Christmas classifies them into four categories: alcoholics and barflies, hustlers and peddlers, the "somewhat straight" (former seamen, retired cab-drivers, pensioners), and "mentals." All in all, they are perceived as a disreputable lot.

The degree to which the manager feels his status to have been contaminated by association with these individuals of questionable position in the social structure is revealed in the complaints he made to me on several occasions. He indicated that he was thinking seriously of quitting the job, as his experiences at the Guinevere were making him hardened, cynical, and sarcastic. Apparently the tenants agreed with his assessment, as they often commented that he had changed, "had to," "at first, he was naïve, friendly to everyone, but now, he knows the score." The tenants, for their part, are quick to find damaging information about the manager's character and past.

Despite the manager's cynical view of the tenants, he does draw distinctions between the transients and the permanent guests, and allows the permanent guests more latitude than the transients. Thus, younger people who are late with the rent will be sent packing, but allowances are made for an elderly permanent, particularly if the individual is a long-term resident, has a history of prompt payment, or has some interesting idiosyncracy of personality that amuses Mr. Christmas. Not only might the manager allow an elderly permanent to stay despite being behind in his rent (in one case, up to three months), he might even tolerate belligerence and a "cussing out" from this recalcitrant tenant. On the other hand, any back talk from a young transient would result in immediate eviction.

The manager shows a certain sympathy for the elderly tenants and stretches the rules for them, particularly in the instance of individuals who catch his fancy. The tenants, for their part, utilize their status as "pets" in a fairly cold-blooded, calculated fashion to derive what benefits they can. Being "in" with the manager has nothing to do with friendship, but a great deal to do with getting something one wants, and is an important coping skill.

The elderly tenants know that the application of hotel policy is often arbitrary and individualistic. An example of this is in the enforcement of the hotel policy to move out tenants if they become nonambulatory. The manager handles these cases on a personal basis; if he likes the person and the individual can work out arrangements to take care of his needs, such as paying a maid to bring food to his room, then Mr. Christmas will most likely allow him to remain. The manager also accepts behavior from the old permanents that he would not tolerate in other tenants: a case in point is the fact that several of the elderly tenants are incontinent and soil their rooms to varying degrees. Conversely, a tenant who Mr. Christmas personally does not like would be evicted with much less reason. In short, the manager wields considerable power, and his power is exercised in a personal and even idiosyncratic manner.

A powerful factor behind the differential treatment accorded the elderly permanents lies not in any particular beneficence on the part of the management, but rather in the practical considerations related to making money out of the hotel's operation. The manager is dependent upon the permanents as surely as they are dependent upon him; they represent a stable source of income that transients do not.[6] The probability of the elderly permanents leaving is remote—they are locked in by their poverty and by their intense desire for privacy and autonomy, which tie them to the depersonalized world of the SRO hotel. It is in this setting that they can realize those needs that characterize their life styles and personal values. Of those who do leave, a large number soon return to the Guinevere. Usually they move to a nearby SRO hotel, but dissatisfaction sets in, and they return to the Guinevere, often requesting the same room. On one occasion, the manager was complaining about an elderly tenant who had "dicked" him out of rent money and left. But, the manager said with a smile, "He'll be back; they all come back sooner or later."

From the point of view of management, elderly tenants present special difficulties in the efficient functioning of the hotel —for example, the high incidence of illness, with the hotel primarily responsible for notifying appropriate services (usual-

6. Shapiro, in a study of nine SROs in New York City, likens slum hotels to privately owned contemporary poorhouses, whose residents are ethnically mixed, socially isolated, poverty-stricken, and beset with physical and mental pathology. She characterizes the relationship between tenants and landlords as one of mutual dependence, colored by a strong element of ambivalence in their attitudes toward one another. Shapiro, "Reciprocal Dependence Between Single-room Occupancy Managers and Tenants."

ly the fire department emergency squad); senility or forget-fulness, resulting in mismanagement of funds and misplaced rent money; vulnerability to being robbed; acting out; and assorted behaviors which interfere with payment of rent. In addition, many of the elderly tenants prefer to be behind in their rent: if they die, they do not want the hotel to make any extra money. The hotel, however, requires payment in advance. Ongoing and rancorous battles are waged over this issue; in fact, with a few of the elderly residents, rent day is a never-ending haggle.

Many tenants do have problems managing their extremely limited resources; some are genuinely forgetful, and not infrequently a drunk old man will be rolled by a prostitute and her pimp. More likely, however, the rent money is not forthcoming because what little money there was has been spent on alcohol or other necessities, or because the individual is attempting to rewrite the hotel rules regarding how much is due and when. The manager has devised an effective scheme to counteract this problem; as the OAA, disability, and social security checks arrive on the first and fifteenth of the month, he makes the individuals endorse and cash them at the desk, paying their rent simultaneously. On occasion, with a particularly recalcitrant individual, the manager refuses to hand over the check until the person agrees to pay. The manager justifies such behavior, which borders on the illegal, by saying that it protects everybody's interests—the hotel's interest because the rent is paid on time and the tenant's interest because he does not lose his room.

However, Mr. Christmas will sometimes go along with persistent offenders, such as the elderly person who has lived at the Guinevere for a number of years, who always eventually pays, whom Mr. Christmas likes, who has not caused trouble. ("Trouble," as defined by the manager, includes such behaviors as "messy" drunkenness, belligerency, homosexuality, fights over women, and "nastiness.") An elderly tenant who falls behind for the first time may be allowed to stay on for a month or two, with the expectation that he will be good for the money.

The manager would not so bend the rules for a young, short-term tenant.

The tenants expect that the manager will maintain a degree of physical protection within the hotel. When trouble occurs, the manager—with his buffer troops of desk clerks, porters, and maintenance men—is expected to take charge and reestablish order. Several policies set down by Mr. Christmas are designed to accomplish this. The manager takes care of emergency situations, such as serious illness, when he has the fire department rescue team there within minutes. Staff people have standing orders to report to him if they have reason to believe that a tenant is ill; and he makes it a habit to call up individuals whom he has not seen around the lobby for a long time. On one occasion the manager strongly upbraided a switchboard operator for unplugging a room because the telephone was off the hook. His orders are to send up a porter in such situations to ascertain that the person is not sick or having a stroke. He was very insistent about this, remarking that one elderly woman who had a heart attack laid in her room for several hours, unable to contact the switchboard.

In the case of a death, the manager notifies survivors, or if no surviving relatives can be reached, arranges for city burial. Potentially violent episodes in the public areas of the hotel are his responsibility, and the tenants expect him to do what is necessary to protect them. The manager routinely deals as a mediator between the tenants and the Department of Social Services.

The utilitarian nature of the relationships between the tenants and the manager is also prototypical of the tenants' transactions with other hotel personnel. They sometimes approach various staff people in order to secure goods, services, or favors —for example, tipping the maid for an extra towel on linen day. A few tenants who are no longer able to get around at all may have to resort to tipping porters and maids to bring them food or toilet articles, but this is very expensive. Many of the maids have been working at the hotel for as long as twenty to twenty-five years. They are predominately black women in their middle years. Everyone attests to their trustworthiness. Infrequently, a tenant who is unable to come up with rent money will claim robbery by one of the maids; however, no one takes the accusation seriously.

The staff members are usually responsive to the tenant's complaints and requests. Toilets are repaired promptly, the exterminator comes every week, linen is clean and delivered on time—although, again, the "pets" are attended to more quickly.

In general, the tenants become involved with hotel staff only to the extent that staff members can do something for them. The pragmatic, impersonal function of such social bonds is rather rigorously demanded. Tenants who are too "familiar" with the hotel employees—for example, asking about their private lives—are behaving in a suspect manner. A polite distance is expected of both parties to the interaction.

In contrast to the relative permanence and reliability of the maids, the desk clerks and switchboard personnel are less reliable and have a rapid turnover. These jobs appear to attract unstable types with histories of trouble and low job stability, and as a rule they do not last long in the Guinevere. During one month, for example, three desk clerks were let go for various reasons. The manager confirmed that one was using his job as a front to pimp women out of the hotel, giving them keys to empty rooms and taking a cut of their earnings; and another individual with a history of violent behavior was arrested for carrying a concealed weapon—while working behind the lobby desk.

Although tenants may approach these employees to obtain services, they do so less readily. Faces change too quickly, and there is less basis for even so skeletal a relationship as that which may be formed with the maids or maintenance people.

CHAPTER THREE

Transients and Permanents

The world of the SRO tenant is a lonely one. People live in physical proximity but for the most part maintain a considerable emotional and social distance from each other. A preliminary view would see little basis for assigning these individuals to social groupings. Their pronounced aloneness is indicative of a world of social isolates and alienated individuals. Nevertheless, there are identifiable groups within the social system of this hotel.

We have seen the first division, which separates the hotel employees from the hotel tenants. The second significant division is the separation of the hotel tenants into two groups—the transients and the elderly permanents (permanent "guests"). The transient tenants are those individuals who have lived in the Guinevere for less than a year, pay by the day or the week, and do not look upon the hotel as their permanent "home."

There exists a definite break between these two groups of tenants, and in almost all ways they constitute separate societies. They rarely have anything to do with each other, and despite their close spatial proximity and overlapping activities (eating at the same restaurants, drinking in the hotel bar, using hotel elevators), they are disinterested in establishing relationships with each other.

A partial explanation for this finding lies in the distinctly negative and resentful attitudes of the permanent guests toward the transients. I encountered no long-term resident who did not clearly distinguish between the transients and the permanent guests. They define transients as intruders. The elderly long-term residents of the Guinevere look upon the hotel as their home, but, in their eyes, the transients merely view the hotel as a place where they can get cheap lodging for a day or a week. There is a strong feeling among the permanents that the transients do not belong there and are interlopers in the private domain of the elderly tenants who have lived in the Guinevere for many years and have every intention of finishing their lives there.

There are significant differences between the transients and the permanents: the transients are considerably younger and were probably born out of the state; they are more likely to be in couples or small family groupings; they spend considerably less time in the hotel (use it primarily as a place to sleep); rarely do they stay longer than a few days or weeks; they do not congregate in the public areas of the hotel for socializing. By contrast, the permanents are elderly; they spend the major portion of their time within the hotel; they are dependent upon the public areas of the hotel for socializing when they desire it; they do not anticipate moving to any other residence; they define the Guinevere as their "home" and, all in all, tend to identify more with the hotel.

The dominant feeling of the elderly permanents is that the transients lower the standards of the hotel. They refer contemptuously to the transients as being on the welfare rolls. They contrast the youth and health of these people with their own advanced years and chronic illnesses, and conclude that being the recipient of state aid is forgivable for themselves, but for "those others," being on the "dole" is a shameful commentary to the effect that "They could work but they don't want to." Several bar fights and near-fights were precipitated by permanents' derogatory remarks to transients, putting them down for receiving welfare. However, the aspect of the transients which the permanents resent most is their behavior. Complaints about the transients disturbing the orderly lives of the permanents and damaging the name of the hotel are common:

> Those others upset the permanent guests. We need privacy, to be left alone. They're, ah, causing trouble. Before you know it, here come the police. He's on the phone, calling the police. Well, he's got to, you see.

> They don't respect nothing, nothing at all, and these here are the worst of the lot.

Thus, the elderly tenants perceive the transients as endangering their own life style by importing into the hotel a variety of bothersome problems, such as drugs, violence, and street rowdies. Their opinion is at least partially shared by the manager, who sees these as the problems that go along with renting to a transient clientele. Of course, he also sees the permanents as generating problems, but different ones. Not surprisingly, the permanents believe that they should receive differential treatment from the hotel management and staff, and, as we have seen, they are supported in this belief by the preferential policies of the manager. Social ties between the transients and permanents are, then, sparse, as the elderly permanents tend to avoid and resent these interlopers in what they define as their home.[1]

Of paramount interest is the degree of interaction and forms of social bonds established among the elderly permanents themselves. The same pattern of minimal, utilitarian-based relational ties is to be found. Close ties between long-term residents are uncommon; intimate relationships are a rarity. The impov-

---

1. The distinction drawn between transients and permanent residents had repercussions for my field work, especially in the early days of the study. My dual role of researcher and transient necessitated the overcoming of both indifference to and ignorance of the goals of the researcher and dislike for the temporary tenant. Whereas the former role became well understood and accepted in the course of the research, the status of transient could at best be neutralized, but not rendered positive.

erished relationships that do develop are sustained on two bases—economic activities and interests, and leisure-time activities and interests.

Because many of these individuals must supplement their meager finances, a significant percentage are more or less continuously seeking a means to earn money. The hotel occasionally has an opening that can be filled by an elderly tenant (however, this is not common), but the most relied upon source of additional income is some variant of "hustling." My use of the term "hustling," or the "hustle," includes several forms of temporary, low-paying, unconventional means of making money that are utilized by tenants in this hotel society. It does not refer only to illegal business activities.[2] Hustling comes in myriad forms in the Guinevere, and ranges from delivering coffee, cigarettes, or liquor ("go-fors"), to selling stolen merchandise, to renting out the back seat of one's car to vagrants, to street vending.

In particular, the street vendors have coalesced into a sizable group with identifying characteristics. The primary source of cohesion is the exigencies that arise in the course of arranging the hustle, with secondary sources of cohesion being generated from the common experiences, interests, and often backgrounds (many have worked previously with carnivals and circuses) that surround hustling. The street vendors are referred to as "carnies" by the tenants, and they enjoy a certain measure of prestige in that they are still working and actively maintaining their independence.

The solidarity that one finds among the carnies is based on the recognition of mutual economic need, and tends to resemble the other relational bonds formed in this hotel society, that is, it tends to be instrumental and nonintimate. The carnies, who may work together eleven hours a day and afterward sit together in the bar drinking, do not consider themselves

2. Chapter 5 treats in depth the importance and pervasiveness of the "hustle" in the lives of the Guinevere tenants.

friends; rather, they define the association as a business partner-ship. When fallings-out occur, and they do occur with predict-able regularity, the cause will be money- or job-related disagree-ments.

The second basis for groupings is the use of leisure time. Most of these people spend the greater part of their time in the hotel. Being retired or semiretired, they, like the old elsewhere in our society, are confronted with a surplus of leisure. The lei-sure activities and interests that head the list at the Guinevere are drinking, betting (the horses and sports events), and social-izing in the public areas of the hotel. Relationships which emerge in the course of these activities are fairly transitory, superficial, and nonintimate. There is much overlapping of re-lationships; it is not feasible to delineate distinct groups, since that would ignore the fluidity of boundaries. Leisure groupings are considerably more evanescent and transitory than the work groups of the carnies.

Leisure time is spent either in one's room, in which case it is not a social affair (with the exception of sexual contacts), or in a public area, in which case it may remain a private activity or may become the stage for interaction. The tenants adhere strictly to the line of demarcation that defines certain areas of the hotel as private and not available for social intercourse, and other areas as public and therefore open to interaction. The most private areas are the residents' rooms. It is rare for anyone to enter but the occupant and the maid. People do not visit each other in their rooms; in fact, the tenants guard the privacy of their rooms with a definiteness that does not bear question.

The supreme importance of their rooms to the tenants is viv-idly demonstrated in the case of one quite elderly man who refused to move from his room on the fifth floor, which had been completely gutted in a fire some months earlier. Despite the almost unlivable condition of his room, he would not move into another. The matter of the room is a source of contention between transients and permanents: the transients are far more likely to invite others to their rooms, occasionally to have small party-like gatherings. Such behavior offends in a profound way the sense of domain of the elderly tenants.

The television room has been defined as only semipublic, and visiting in this room is a risky business. The presence of television is of minimal influence, as many of the elderly residents come and sit for hours with the television off, and little or no interaction will take place.

Visiting and socializing properly occur in those areas of the hotel that the tenants define as public, and takes the form of congregating in these areas, such as the lobbies, the front stoop, or the Guinevere restaurant at 7:30 A.M. On warm evenings, small groups will gather on the front stoop; during the afternoon and evening, two or three people can be observed drinking together in the bar; the lobbies are always available to anyone who wishes to spend some time standing and watching as people come and go.

There is some visiting with residents of nearby hotels, although generally they are avoided, as they are believed to be of lower class. These visits will take place in a restaurant, or perhaps in nearby Lower Park, or in the lobby of the Guinevere. It is less likely that a tenant of the Guinevere will visit someone in another hotel. During warm weather, there is a fair amount of street activity—walking down to Eddie's Restaurant or the Park, standing on the front stoop, and the like. Wherever the visiting and socializing may occur, the interaction conforms to a rigid pattern of racial, sexual, and even hotel segregation.

The topics of conversation most often center around events at the hotel—indeed, the tenants display a lively interest in happenings at the hotel that immediately and routinely affect them. Among the men, the principal subjects of interest are betting, drinking, sex, and the hustle. Checking up on each other commands a major share of the conversation. Thus, it is noted when a tenant is untidy or unshaven, or in some way looks as if he or she is deteriorating. They note any deviation from the normal in either dress or behavior. It is popular to make comparisons that are favorable to oneself. Gossip is pervasive and there are no loyalties. There are, in fact, frequent fallings-out over gossip that gets back to the target. There are some vendettas of several years' standing which originated over gossip. Danger is also a favorite topic, danger as personified in the black—the black addict, the black mugger, the black rapist —the fear of blacks permeates the conversations of these people.

Betting is another favorite pastime of the men and a lively source of conversation. The bets are small—rarely over two dollars—and are handled by "Jerry the Bookie," an elderly man who has lived in the hotel for years and who rents a small office in the hotel lobby. Jerry is respected by his patrons; he handles things in a businesslike fashion and does not cheat them. Occasionally, men from the hotel may go to the track together, but it is a matter of convenience. Despite the fact that betting is ubiquitous and a source of endless debate, friendships are not likely to develop around this common interest.

The hotel bar is the scene of much visiting among the elderly tenants. During the weekdays and nights, most of the bar crowd consists of Guinevere residents; on the weekends, there are more outsiders. Some of the elderly men drink there on a daily basis; some drink alone, others have drinking companions. These drinking companions part company outside the bar; their friendship does not survive outside the common interest of drinking. There is a demonstrable rhythm to the drinking—more drinking for perhaps four or five days at the first of the month, and then tapering off as the check is used up.

The bar is an important center for many of the business deals of the carnies—hustles are arranged, and money transactions are numerous. The bar is a kind of crossroads for carnies, not only from the Guinevere but from the whole area, and on occasion the bar crowd may be composed mainly of carnies.

Finally, the bar is the setting for sexual contacts. Prostitutes from the area work the men in the bar, particularly on the first and fifteenth of the month, when there is an influx of "hookers." They disappear in a few days, having skimmed off the top of residents' checks.

Although the bar is a natural area for interaction and is often full of pairs and small groups in lively conversation, at all times a good proportion of the drinkers will be sitting alone and, if approached by others, will be quite as likely to respond in a surly fashion as a receptive one. The fact is that a major portion of the activities of these people is carried out alone: they eat alone; they go walking alone; many drink alone. They do not telephone each other; they do not visit in each others' rooms; they do not commemorate special occasions, such as birthdays, holidays, deaths.

Looking at the society of these elderly people, one is forcefully struck by the pervasive strictures against attempting to become too intimate with one another. They do not encourage relationships that permit mutual concern or the sharing of deeply personal matters. It is common for them to say that there are no real friendships in the Guinevere:

> I don't have any friends, *real* friends here. I don't get too thick because they'll be prying into my business.

> If you get friendly with them, they start tellin' you about their problems and I don't want to hear it.

> Nobody's friends. Why, they'd give a dollar to a prossie than to one who thinks he's a friend and needs it.

> Listen, the only one here everybody talks to is Jerry [the bookmaker].

As for mutual aid, there are occasional instances of it; but in general, the tenants' belief that one could be sick for days and maybe even die without anyone knowing or caring about it is an accurate appraisal. I heard reports of several elderly individuals who had died in their rooms and been found there days later by the maids. Even individuals who interact more or less frequently with each other become psychologically unavailable when confronted with the option of moving toward a closer, more demanding relationship. Several people summed up the situation by remarking that "It's everyone for himself."

The dominant values of privacy and autonomy operate to inhibit the formation of deeply personal or enduring relationships. Behavior that reflects contradictory assumptions is met with reactions ranging from suspicion to icy aloofness to alarm. Real intimacy is not expected or encouraged, even among tenants who have lived on the same floor for years. This avoidance of close ties extends in at least two cases to close family. There are two brothers living in the hotel who never talk and have never acknowledged their relationship. When an elderly woman died, it was discovered that her sister lives in the hotel. They had not talked or interacted for at least the eight years that they had been there.

Related to the pattern of avoiding close relationships is the mutual suspicion the tenants display toward one another. To put it as succinctly as possible, in this society of the alone, suspicion is institutionalized. The avoidance of intimate contacts is related to the taken-for-granted meanings that attach to their identification of each other as untrustworthy characters, who will use any person who is not cautious and wary. It is taken for granted that the actions of the other are suspect and that any apparently selfless motive is undoubtedly concealing the real motive.

The routinizing of suspicion is facilitated by the presence of a hotel "mystique"—a core of commonly held beliefs about the supposed "type" that lives in hotels. These people are more than casually aware of the low repute in which their class is held. In addition, the group includes a sizable number who have had, at best, checkered careers, often involving petty crime, psychiatric treatment, indigence. In short, their personal biographies reflect their failure in varying degrees to fulfill cultural and social mandates. A consequence of this knowledge is the ubiquity of face-saving maneuvers. The most widely used technique for saving face is the remaking of personal history. Thus, one is never certain whether the story the other is telling is true or manufactured for the audience. Not surprisingly, attitudes of cynicism and suspicion predominate. These people, in their need to conceal and refurbish, must jealously guard their own secrets, and yet be realistically cynical about the stories of others, who presumably are doing the same reconstructing of their pasts. Although this suspicion pervades many aspects of the ways in which they do (and do not) relate to one another, it is nowhere more manifest than in their routine assumption that everyone has something to hide and that, consequently, most explanations of background are false. As a core belief of the mystique, everyone is there for a "reason," and this "reason" probably is something reprehensible. Thus it is to be expected that if one is so imprudent as to inquire about backgrounds, fabrications will be in order. It is considered rude to inquire about another's past. When, on a rare occasion, an account is offered, the listener is expected to act as if he believes it.

The insistence upon independence can even involve the denial of relationships that are functional and operative. Thus, one carny "boss" repeatedly asserted that he worked alone, when in fact he always worked with two or three helpers. Yet he displayed considerable pride in the fact that he "doesn't work with anybody," and denied any dependency.

The coming together of independence and mutual distrust is vividly revealed in the words of an eighty-year-old widow: "I take care of me, because no one else is going to. I don't trust anybody. I look for the angle. I tabulate them and then I get their number. It's best to keep them guessing, then to go whining and crying, oh, like, to the manager."

In the face of accumulating losses—physical, mental, social, and financial—these elderly people sustain a determined autonomy and a fierce sense of privacy. Their mode of adjustment means that they pay a heavy price in terms of social isolation; many of them identify loneliness as one of the generic features of old age, certainly their old age:

> The biggest problem of old people anywhere in the world is loneliness. Yes, I could show you how old, re-

tired men go from bar to bar because they haven't anything to do, anywhere to be, anybody who cares.

It's [the hotel] full of strangers who come and go. I shared the bath with this man. Never saw him for three months. Then, one night, his room caught on fire. It was the first time I ever saw him. It's very lonely, especially for the women.

Notwithstanding the admission of the pains of loneliness, the overwhelming evidence of this study supports the finding that these people avoid relationships. Isolation and loneliness is a price that they are prepared to pay to maintain their independence. Theirs is a world of the alone, a world that they have partially made and, at any rate, are sustaining. The situated features of the hotel mitigate against building viable interpersonal ties. These people have limited resources that reduce their capacity to make the compromises needed to sustain intimate relationships. Relationships are nonintimate and instrumental, and serve mainly as vehicles for getting what one needs. There is a merging of situational (social) and individual (psychological) forces which gives shape to and maintains this atomistic society of aged.

CHAPTER FOUR

Adaptive Strategies

An account of this society of aged residents of an SRO hotel would be incomplete without an examination of the means they use to satisfy routine needs, ranging from the basic biological necessities to maintain health, have adequate shelter, eat meals, secure safety, and the like, to the higher needs that give rise to ego-enhancing activities. It is a sociological commonplace that groups develop characteristic routines of role relationships that become institutionalized as "normal" modes of adjustment. These modes of adjustment facilitate the overall ability of the group to maintain itself, and permit individual members to satisfy personal needs. To support these routine adjustment behaviors, certain attitudes and expectancies are also institutionalized and are elaborated into a dense, if frequently covert, network of taken-for-granted meanings, which serve not only to define contextual reality but also to delineate effective and permissible coping skills.

The elaboration of effective coping skills is necessary for the survival of the group, as it provides for the continued ability of individuals to maintain adequate adjustment modes in relation to the contingencies of their environment. The primary burden of affixing taken-for-granted meanings (definitions of situations) is the attendant conservation of resources by the individuals. Thus, all activity need not wait until a complicated process of defining and "figuring out" occurs; rather, the individual can plug the taken-for-granted meanings into a specific situation, and conserve energy for situations of a more problematic character.

Initially, I conceived this aspect of the Guinevere tenants' life style as falling into two separate categories: (1) coping skills and adaptive stratagems utilized to meet routine needs, and (2) special or emergency coping skills required to meet those problematic situations which tend to fall outside the realm of the routine. However, it became more and more apparent that for this group of people such a distinction might be misleading. For these people, the routine overlaps so markedly with the problematic that providing for basic needs is never assured, never entirely routinized.

The aged tenants of the Guinevere are little different from other groups of people in seeking to establish a minimum of stability and order so as to accomplish the tasks that are indigenous to human communities everywhere, namely, survival, goals, allocation of resources, meaning and value, control, security. The order and stability that must be obtained come harder to the residents of the Guinevere: the world of the slum-hotel dweller is an attenuated one. As we have seen, it is a world of strangers who come and go, who live in close physical proximity but erect strong barriers to social and psychological closeness. It is a world where cynicism and suspicion are ubiquitous, where reliance and intimacy are scarce indeed. It is a world that is surrounded by the extremes of human alienation, cruelty, and despair: it may be a world that is in fundamental ways antagonistic to the humane survival of people.

The tenants in the Guinevere are further attenuated in that they are aging and aged, and they, as a group, have reduced resources to cope with their environment. They suffer from declining health, sometimes decreasing mental acuity, reduced mobility, and the accompanying difficulties of allocating extremely limited resources, economic and personal, to take care of both routine and extraordinary needs and events.

Within this context, the Guinevere permanents have articulated a system of coping strategies that serve them well. Behaviors that might appear "pathological" or indicative of "poor adjustment" in a different context, constitute viable means of adaptation and survival in their world of meanings. The reasons for their avoidance of close relationships and the trust and vulnerability which result from such forms of interaction, the reasons for their extreme isolation, will elude us if we fall back on simplistic explanations—that is, if we assume that their lack of sociability is an inevitable function of the aging process. To understand their insistence upon privacy, independence, and anonymity, their nonchalance and insensitivity toward illness and death of their colleagues, their preoccupation with violence, we must enter into their world of taken-for-granted meanings and thereby come to identify the situated aspects of their conduct.[1]

As has been stated, one goal of my research was to develop an extensive descriptive analysis of the social world of this group, with special attention to the degree and intensity of social interaction. An issue of secondary interest in the original formulation of this research was that of identifying the role of deviance in the life styles of these elderly slum residents, and of locating mechanisms utilized to combat and control deviance. As the study progressed, this secondary issue came to assume a greater prominence. This occurred as the data turned my attention to its crucial part in understanding a variety of behaviors. Deviance—from the troublesomely unpredictable to the catastrophically violent—assumes a major role in the world of these aged SRO tenants. Lionized in current sociology, the issue of deviant behaviors is a stark reality for these people, and it shapes both their attitudes toward each other and their expectations pertinent to behavior.

1. I am arguing against a sociology of *aging* behavior in favor of a sociology which grounds all behaviors to specific situations, and defines these behaviors as forms of adaptive strategies to manipulate, give meaning to, and derive value from the particular environment.

The survival stratagems utilized by these people are inextricably linked to the ever-present threat of deviance, which in various forms surrounds these people and perpetually threatens to engulf them. A fundamental mechanism for the control of deviance is their avoidance of close relationships.

These people do not (and probably cannot) control deviance emanating both from the "outside" and from within their midst, but they attempt to avoid it by so restricting and constraining their ties to and dependencies upon others as to minimize the effects of deviance on their own lives. These effects include the high probability that close relationships will become exploitative associations; the constant threat of violence; and the reciprocal norms of distrust and suspicion. It is time to consider coping behaviors, their relationship to needs and deviancy, and the linkage to characteristic forms of social interaction.

NEEDS AND COPING STRATEGIES

Life at the Guinevere has its discernible rhythms. Rent is due; room-cleaning day arrives; the checks come in; there are nightly brawls and street fights; there is an increased number of deaths during the holidays and spring months. One cluster of factors contributing to the rhythm is the necessity to attend to needs. Needs must be met, ways must be found to keep body and soul together. A factor that distinguishes this society from many others in our affluent culture is the greater effort and time which these people must expend to satisfy day-to-day needs. Those goods and services that many of us take for granted—such as nutritious and appealing meals, attractive and comfortable housing, money in our pockets, good health— are rarely assumed by the tenants at the Guinevere.[2]

One of the most serious reasons why these people fail to meet

2. Lawton and Kleban, "The Aged Resident of the Inner City," found significant differences between SRO aged and the aged in the general population. For the SRO elderly, all available energy and resources are continually being mustered to cope with the most fundamental needs of survival.

basic needs is their extremely limited financial assets. Eighty percent receive some form of state aid; few have any savings. A minority are on small pensions, supplemented by social security. The average monthly income is below $200; from this sum, an average of $82.36 is paid for rent. This leaves approximately $117.64 to meet other needs through the month. The severe limitation of funds which can be allocated to pay for food, transportation, medical expenses, and so forth, has identifiable consequences. Many of the needs are not met; prosthetic devices are not purchased; meals are inadequate and do not fulfill the greater protein requirements of elderly persons; medical needs are left unattended. The mass exodus of tenants, many of whom have lived in the Guinevere for years, when the owners raised the rent two dollars a month, is a reminder of the unalterable reality of drastically circumscribed funds. It is a standing joke that the first day of the month is the day everyone waits for. If one of the old people stops anticipating the mailman's arrival, then chances are he is about gone.[3]

One fundamental need whose satisfaction requires a considerable output of energy and resources is meals. There are no cooking facilities or refrigerators in the rooms. For the most part, the tenants must eat out at nearby restaurants, which imposes numerous hardships: the food is expensive, and going out on a regular basis increases the risk of being robbed and mugged, and demands a physical effort for these people, many of whom are not well. The toll extracted increases during the winter months as the weather worsens. Nevertheless, the majority of the elderly tenants eat at one of the three nearby restaurants.

There are two restaurants within walking distance, the "Griddle Shop" and the "Boulevard Cafe." The Guinevere Res-

---

3. It is one thing to consider in the abstract the hardships of living on $117.64 a month, and quite another to attempt to do so. I tried to live on this pittance but failed miserably. For those colleagues who lament the "soft" nature of participant observation, I can only say that an empty stomach is far more enlightening than any number of coded questionnaires.

taurant is attached to the hotel itself. All are dirty and smell of urine. To reach the Griddle Shop and the Boulevard Cafe one must walk down streets out of which several narrow alleys lead, and access to them is often accomplished at a considerable risk to these vulnerable individuals. The Guinevere Restaurant is physically safer to reach, but its prices are higher than the other two restaurants. The tenants may go there to sit and have coffee, tea, or soup, but they do not make a habit of purchasing meals there. The Griddle Shop issues meal tickets and has the lowest prices; unfortunately, the tenants are for the most part fearful of patronizing this restaurant, as it is sandwiched between two apartment buildings that house mostly blacks. The tenants of the Guinevere have often been victimized and brutalized by occupants of these two buildings, and they are understandably reluctant to run the risk. The Boulevard Cafe accepts food stamps and allows credit, keeping a running tab; it does not discriminate against those on state aid. The Guinevere does not accept food stamps, and has a large sign by the cash register that reads, "NO CREDIT." However, the owners do occasionally extend credit to individuals who have been coming there for years and are "in" with one of the owners.

Most of the elderly tenants prefer to eat at either the Boulevard Cafe or the Guinevere. Because of its cheaper prices and larger portions, the Boulevard is where the dinner meal is more likely to be eaten. In addition, there is a feeling that the owners do more to accommodate their elderly patrons, as they carry foods these people request, such as Jello or fruit. Typically, the more expensive Guinevere Restaurant collects a large number of elderly tenants in the early morning hours; they come and sit for long periods, drinking coffee and eating a piece of toast, listening and watching the other customers.

The well-known "tea and toast syndrome" of the aged is prevalent among these people. Many have a deficient diet, and hunger is not uncommon. Generally, they eat one meal a day. They often have no set time for that meal, only taking care to go early enough to return before dark, thus recognizing the ever-present element of danger. The daily meal is often hardly sufficient to warrant the name, sometimes consisting of coffee, toast, soup, and jello. A meal that includes meat and vegetables is a treat. The following field-note entry is illustrative:

> While sitting in the Boulevard, waiting for the waitress to bring my order, I observed an elderly white-haired woman whom I had often seen in the TV room. She was apparently having quite a session with the waitress. She asked the waitress several times if the meat was tender and referred to the three entrees listed in the menu. The waitress grew impatient and abruptly assured her that everything was good and that the spare ribs were especially tender. The white-haired woman did not seem satisfied but continued to inquire as to the condition of the meat. The waitress left, saying that she would bring the spare rib dinner. The woman spoke to the back of the departing waitress, saying that she only ate meat once a week and she wanted to be sure it was tender. I looked at my own plate of Salisbury steak and felt ashamed.

Meals are expensive, involve a definite effort, and demand certain real risks and hardships for these people. That they do not eat enough is understandable, given the situational factors that stand in the way.

There are alternative ways of meeting this need. Some buy lunchmeat and bread at the nearby market and make sandwiches to eat in their rooms, the "lunchmeat and mayonnaise" crowd, according to one desk clerk. A very few have hot plates. In a pinch, one can turn an iron upside down between two Gideon Bibles. One or two have even purchased styrofoam coolers to preserve food, thereby reducing the frequency with which they have to go to the market (ice is provided free in the lobby). However, those who prepare their meals in their rooms must, for the most part, purchase their food daily. This requires a considerable effort, and, in addition, the market is expensive and carries inferior goods. This is, of course, typical of supermarkets in ghetto areas; furthermore, this market routinely exploits these elderly poor. When they use food stamps to purchase goods, the owners skim off the top; thus, one gets five dollars' worth of merchandise for ten dollars in food stamps. Toward the end of the month, as people become more desperate, the store skims off more.

Only a small number cook regularly on hot plates in their rooms; they are most likely to resort to this when they run out of money and are unable to eat at a restaurant. Some cannot put aside the money to buy a hot plate and so they join the "lunchmeat and mayonnaise" group. The drinkers can, for the most part, dispense with food; they prefer to "drink their meals." For them, running out of money means borrowing enough to buy some cheap wine, so that they can "hide out" in their rooms and await the next check. Cheap muscatel has replaced "squeeze" as the low-cost drink for the lean times. "Squeeze" is made by pouring canned heat (Sterno) into a sock or pillowcase, squeezing the alcohol into a jar, and diluting it with water. Fortunately, the practice is falling into disuse as the price of Sterno outdistances that of the cheapest wines.

Whether it involves a daily trek to a nearby restaurant to purchase cottage cheese and Jello or living on lunchmeat sandwiches, this routine and commonplace act becomes an ordeal for these people, requiring a disproportionate outlay of both economic and physical resources. The conjunction of scarce funds and their physical vulnerability serves to render so basic and mundane an activity problematic.

Behaviors associated with meals are rather dull when compared to the richness of activities that develop around the issue of paying rent. There is an inevitability about rent day, and yet these elderly tenants have access to a remarkable array of strategies designed to delay, deny, and redefine both the time and the amount of payment.

Of the many reasons why paying rent is a problematic issue, the most prominent are insufficient funds and lack of agreement between management and tenant about when the rent is due and how much is due. In a population such as this, people often have difficulty budgeting their meager monies in order to meet such a basic expense as rent. Even when money is well budgeted, emergencies do occur, robberies are common, misplaced funds are not unknown. However, the most common source of disagreement over the issue of rent results from differing expectations. The manager expects his tenants to pay on time, and his understanding of "on time" means "in advance." Those who receive social security normally pay by the month, those on state aid, biweekly. The tenants, on the other hand, want to pay by the week: they see it as less expensive, less money going out at one time. Also, they define "on time" as payment *after* the service is rendered, that is, they want to be a week *behind* in their rent, they insist upon this. Constant battles are waged over this issue of the time that the rent is due; indeed, there are some elderly tenants who go through shouting matches with the manager twice a month and have been doing so for years.

The manager defines the rent monies as his. When one elderly man, who was receiving a certain amount from social services for his rent, moved into a cheaper room, the manager was indignant and stated quite forcefully, "That's *my* money." He threatened to expose the tenant to the agency unless he moved back to the more expensive room.

Nonpayment of rent has reliable consequences. The transient who fails to pay is contacted by the manager. Either he pays up or he is evicted, and the hotel keeps the luggage until payment is made. In the case of an elderly permanent resident, the manager has his room "plugged." A small metal device is inserted into the lock of the door so that the key cannot be used to unlock the door, and the tenant loses access to his room. The tenants bitterly resent plugging; no other action or policy on the part of hotel personnel so outrages them. Tenants whose rooms are plugged—and there are a number to whom this happens with predictable regularity—become righteous martyrs and receive considerable verbal support and sympathy from the other tenants. That they may be several days or even weeks behind in their rent is deemed insufficient cause to treat them so poorly. The following statements are typical responses to the outrage of being plugged:

> Well, I'm sure plugging's uncalled for. We're permanent guests and are always good for the money.

> We keep this hotel running. Our money pays the bills. They're depending on us old-timers! They need us. He [the manager] just plugs everybody some days. It's wrong. He needs our business and he knows it.

Some tenants anticipate being plugged and have stratagems to forestall it. The most often used ploy is the "con." Similar to the use of conning in manufacturing a personal history, the conning of the manager consists of an act and a convincing story designed to justify the fact that one is behind with the rent. The act may include other hotel employees if the tenant presents his "case" to them and requests that they "mention it" to the manager. The content of the con ranges from denial of being in arrears ("I'm sure that I already paid"), to indignation ("I always pay on time!"), to threats (accompanied by shouts and profanity), to sincere promises to pay, to the myriad versions of how the money has been lost or stolen, and "Could I just have a little more time?" On occasion, tenants will turn on the picture of helplessness and pitiful old age to add a convincing dimension to their battery of excuses. The list of excuses is endless, and ranges from claims of having been robbed, to the plea that an anticipated check has not arrived.

When the con fails and excuses can no longer forestall reprisals—in short, when plugging is imminent—the tenant may resort to a more extreme tactic. He may lock himself inside his room and refuse to come out or to answer his telephone. If his key is in the lock on the inside, the door cannot be plugged. This strategy is relatively effective, in that it can delay things for a few days at least. The manager waits it out, periodically sending up porters and desk clerks to knock on the door and issue threats. Eventually, the tenant has to come out, by which time he is usually willing to settle the dispute. Even in the unusual case where the rent still is not paid, the tenant can manage to avoid losing a place to sleep. One elderly woman who was six weeks behind in her rent was plugged, and for the next two weeks she slept in a chair in the television room.

No shame or stigma attaches to the individual whose room is plugged. Whatever the circumstances pertaining to and resulting in plugging, the reaction of the tenants is unanimous: plugging is wrong; the tenant has the right to feel aggrieved. This action should not be taken against a permanent resident. This opinion is often held simultaneously with the knowledge that the tenant's excuse was most likely a con. He probably does owe rent, but that is only because the manager has a perverse idea of the time and amount of money due. Furthermore, the other tenants do not find fault on the part of the delinquent because he is a permanent resident. That the particular tenant may be a chronic offender carries little weight. As far as they are concerned, the manager is guilty of cupidity: after all, the permanents are always "good for it," and they ought not to be treated like someone who has just walked in off the street.

Plugging denies one of the most crucial assumptions held by the individuals in this society—the privacy and sacrosanct character of their rooms. It is an affront to their insistence that these rooms are their homes and sanctuaries. For any permanent tenant, plugging cannot be justified; strategies employed to avoid it may range from the furtive to the unrealistic, but all are understandable from their point of view.

An underlying factor that influences the ability of these people to manage in their setting is the status of their health. Disabilities and handicaps abound. In addition, they are susceptible to falls and injuries. More pertinent to our understanding of their behavior is their attitude toward these various physical and mental handicaps. The tenuous status of their health constitutes a major source of anxiety for them. They equate illness with old age: infirmity is the essence of old age.

To maintain reasonably good health is to keep at bay old age with its implications of dependency.[4] An elderly man who still works as a street vendor summed up his feelings: "Nobody cares about the old. Put them in nursing homes and they don't have the strength to fight it. But the problem, real problem is health. Everybody deteriorates. You're old when you feel it. A lot of old people want to die, just waiting to die. It's because of their infirmities. The sicknesses wear you down, make you feel old." These people define losses in physical and mental well-being as powerfully threatening events that may result in the loss of independence and the erosion of all that they value. This pervasive fear leads to a continual interest in drawing comparisons, in checking up on one's own mental and physical competencies by contrasting them with the sometimes visible and rapid decline of other aged tenants in the hotel. They fear mental deterioration more acutely than physical illness, for they believe that mental decline is a catastrophic event that will bring about the destruction of those values that characterize their life style—independence, privacy, freedom.

Little concern is manifested over the possibility of death; their concern is with life and with the threats, such as illness, that would severely attenuate life. The tenants meet the frequent emergencies at the Guinevere with a singular nonchalance. On the average, at least one aged tenant dies a month, and strokes and near-deaths are common. When a death does occur, the tenants give it little notice.

The tenants' lack of involvement with dying behaviors is in contrast to various dying behaviors exhibited by hotel staff. The manager takes care of all arrangements: he contacts the medical examiner; he gets in touch with survivors, and where there are none, notifies the city. It is typically the manager

4. The literature is replete with studies that reveal the intimate association between poor health and self-definitions of being "old." See Preston, "Subjectively Perceived Agedness and Retirement"; Schwartz and Kleemeier, "The Effects of Illness and Age upon Some Aspects of Personality"; and Streib, "Morale of the Retired."

who writes "finis" to the story of the elderly tenant who dies in the hotel. If the tenant dies in the hospital or the ambulance, the manager has arranged the place of death. Other hotel personnel play roles in the management of death. The hotel maid is usually the one who discovers the body, and this fact has given rise to at least one bit of hotel mythology. The maids claim that they know when a tenant has died before they enter his room; they claim that they can smell death. An interesting economic feature of dying behaviors in the Guinevere is that the time that elapses between the death of a tenant and the discovery of his body is usually dependent upon the price of the room. This is due to the fact that the price of the room is related to how often the maids come.

The involvement of tenants in the management of death is minor. They typically do not find the body; they do not attend funerals (and do not expect others to attend their own). They little note the death of one of their colleagues unless the person in question was a real "character" or died in some particularly horrible or violent fashion. One of the few behaviors associated with the management of death that these people articulate has to do with their defining of the "about to die." Tenants who seem to be deteriorating very rapidly may be spoken of as terminal cases. In one instance, an elderly alcoholic who entered into a marathon bout of drinking that immediately preceded, and in all likelihood precipitated, his death, was defined by the other tenants as "an about to die." To a large extent he was, in fact, socially defined as dead, and no further references were made to him, except in the past tense. His actual death, a week later, drew little notice or comment.

DEVIANCE AND DANGER

A Guinevere resident offered me the following advice: "What you do is, don't take no purse with you. When you go out, take a dollar or so, what you can take to lose. 'Cause they'll steal, for sure, so don't carry more'n you can afford to part with, but don't go out with nothing. They might get mad, 'cause you don't have something and they're mean, and they'll beat you up anyway, for not having any money to give them."

Danger is a dominant theme in the lexicon of fears. All of the tenants' activities are, to some extent, influenced by their own perception of the ever-present possibility of danger. In their relationship to their environment and in the ways in which they cope, they are forced to tailor their activities to meet the exigencies of an environment that can be described as nonsupportive, even hostile.

Deviance in its myriad forms is endemic to the area, with its high concentration of social and psychological pathology. All of these slum dwellers are acutely aware of the possibility that an innocent-appearing situation might culminate in their own victimization or exploitation. The fear is there; long-term residents report that it never entirely disappears—going up in the elevator with a stranger, somebody behind them in one of those dark, narrow hallways. Particularly, it is the fear of physical violence that dominates the lives and adjustment stratagems of these aged occupants. Everyone agrees on at least one issue— the area in which they live is exceedingly dangerous. Many attribute this to the high proportion of blacks in the neighborhood. Some blame it on the widespread usage of illegal drugs. Whatever their beliefs as to the forces behind it, all are continuously and pervasively concerned with violence and their own perceived vulnerability. As a consequence, the specter of danger is a compelling force in the organization of their life styles and affects the nature of their social relationships.

Their preoccupation with danger and violence is not without substantial basis. During the first two months of field work, the following events occurred within the hotel: an elderly man was the victim of an armed robbery, there were three beatings, a woman was thrown out of a sixth-floor window, a tenant was gunned down by police officers in the lobby, a recently released mental patient threatened tenants with a loaded gun, at least half a dozen elderly tenants were roughed up by pimps, and several fights and near-fights occurred in the bar.

All of these elderly can relate experiences in which they felt that their lives were in immediate danger. The following two episodes capture the feelings of being vulnerable in hostile surroundings:

> I was going to my room on the ninth floor, and two others, they live in the hotel, were in it [the elevator], too. We heard sounds, like fighting, like people fighting. Sounded like they was falling against the elevator door. It was the seventh floor. Everyone did the same thing, we jumped back against the wall and said, "push the button," meaning we'd better go back down to the lobby. But no one did it. So, it opened at the seventh floor, and two men are fighting. They're just young men, and one lives in the hotel—he's a veteran. I've seen him at the desk. I think the other lives over at the Benson. They were fighting and the one was bleeding. He looked at me and said, "What are you looking at, old man?" But I didn't say anything to him. They went on fighting. The man, the one in the blue shirt, pushed it, and we went down to the lobby, and I was thinking the whole way, yes, just a god-damn jungle we're living in, down here.

> Two of 'em come into the lobby, and they was black and mouthy. I knew they was trouble, looking for it. But I was over by the door and couldn't get to the elevator or maybe the TV room because I'd had to walk right in front of the one, and sure, they was looking for trouble. Right away, they started gettin' smart with Blackstock [the desk clerk]. The manager come out and talked to them. But they wanted trouble. The one especially was shooting off his mouth about how he would hate to wipe out all these innocent people. I went on the side of the cigarette machine, so if he started to snooting, I'd have a place to duck down. I think he [the manager] handled it all right, talked to them polite, and after, they left. But the one said he'd be back. That's what you get when you let "niggers" in.

Beatings and robberies are commonplace in this area, and these people are likely targets.[5] There is little surprise expressed when such events occur. For many of them, leaving the hotel is a major event and fraught with personal danger. It is a common practice to pin their money to the insides of their clothes; women do not carry handbags on the streets. They agree that the best policy is to venture out of the hotel only when necessary, and then select the best time of the day. They avoid some streets; for example, they do not walk down Main Street to get to the downtown shopping center. They claim that there are too many young black men who hang about the corners and hassle them.[6]

The front stoop of the hotel attracts a sizable number of local toughs, who hang out around the hotel and nearby bars. They occasionally harass and frighten the elderly tenants. The manager attempts to reassure his tenants and avoid confrontation by periodically chasing them away. A short time prior to the beginning of this study, the manager had the porters remove several chairs from the lobby. Meant for the tenants, they had been usurped by street hoods who terrorized the tenants who attempted to sit in them. He has further attempted to reduce the incidence of beatings and robberies inside the hotel (which occur in the elevators, the hallways, and the rooms) by issuing strict orders to his staff to keep alert to the presence of nonresidents in the hotel. This order is obeyed rigorously, especially if a black person enters the hotel lobby or bar. He is watched closely, approached and questioned, and, with little cause, asked to leave. The manager has a firm policy with regard to blacks in the bar: they are kept waiting, with the barmaids and

5. Lawton and Kleban, in two studies of an SRO in Philadelphia, found that the aged tenants were prime targets for purse-snatching, armed robbery, mugging, and burglary. The authors concluded that the need for and inability to realize physical security underlay the aged tenants' failure to gain satisfaction of other needs. Lawton and Kleban, "Aged Residents"; Lawton, Kleban, and Singer, "The Aged Jewish Person and the Slum Environment."

6. During my residence in the Guinevere, the tenants continually instructed me as to what to do and what not to do in order to avoid dangerous situations.

bartenders carefully ignoring them, until they either leave or cause a scene, at which time, of course, the police are called. Tenants who make the mistake of drinking with a black are banned from the bar for twenty-four hours and ostracized by other tenants.

The threat of victimization and violence can originate not only from the outside, but also from individuals within the hotel. There are instances of hotel personnel attempting to exploit these elderly people. A retired nurse related the following episode:

> I left my room to do some shopping. I had received my check that morning and Kelly [the desk clerk] cashed it for me. Well, he was still on duty as I left to pick up some small things down at the dime store. I went about a block and then I remembered I had forgotten, oh, something, and I returned to the hotel. When I entered my room, I realized that my door was unlocked, and I was sure that I had locked it. But it wasn't linen day, so it couldn't have been one of the maids. I had a hunch, you see, so, I went out into the hall, and I didn't see anybody. But, I noticed that the door to the janitor's closet was ajar. I opened it and found a young woman crouching down. Well, I knew right away, then. She shoved me aside and ran down the hall and down the stairway. When she pushed me aside, she dropped the key, and it was, it was the pass key to my room. So, you see, that was the plan, the desk clerk knew that I had cashed my check just that morning, so, he was setting me up for a rip-off. But I didn't go to the manager, oh no, I decided to handle this matter myself. I took the pass key back to the desk clerk, and said "Listen here, bub, I know just what you're up to, and if anything ever happens again, I'll go right to the police." Oh yes, he knew I meant business.

It is strongly believed that another source of trouble is the transients. Family feuds are not uncommon among these younger tenants, and altercations sometimes spill over into the halls and lobbies. Also, the elderly tenants associate these "outsiders" with "pill-popping" and loud parties, which can culminate in fights and calls for the police. In short, they define them as contributing to the bad name of the hotel and adding to the dangers and problems with which the permanent resident has to cope.

The resentment and fear of the many kinds of deviance and violence to be found in the environment of these people is tempered in their reactions to similarly undesirable forms of behavior originating in their own midst. There is a significant amount of deviance displayed by some of the elderly tenants, and various kinds of acting out are common. Behavior that would elicit condemnation and intolerance if exhibited by an outsider may, on the other hand, be tolerated in one of the elderly permanents. I witnessed several instances in which the permanents were tolerant toward and unshocked by behaviors of other permanent residents that clearly manifested psychosis. They admit that the behavior is eccentric, even shameful, but at the same time they would not suggest the removal of the offender. Even extremely bizarre behaviors are tolerated from a permanent resident; much less markedly deviant behavior on the part of a transient would elicit indignation and complaints. Their response to the following exhibition put on by an elderly permanent resident is instructive:

> Josephine has lived in the hotel for several years and works part-time as a baby-sitter and domestic. Today she put on a show for everyone to see. On her way to the hotel, she was lifting her dress above her head and saying suggestive things to people on the street. She came into the hotel lobby and continued to expose herself, interspersing her suggestive comments with profanity. She was masturbating openly and continued to beckon to some of the men who were standing in the lobby. After some time, at least fifteen minutes, the desk clerk had the switchboard operator, an elderly woman, take Josephine up to her room. The aftermath was that

there was some talk that Josephine was a harmless thing and that she was "nuts" and that her behavior didn't do any harm to anybody. Besides, "she has worked hard all her life and has had a rough time of it."

The elderly tenants react to such violations of "normal" behavioral standards with a certain imperturbability mixed with a denial that the Guinevere has as many "weirdos" as the other hotels in the area. Another tenant being beaten and robbed or a black coming into the hotel will stir up more concern than any number of spectacles such as the psychotic woman in the lobby. Their tolerance of such behaviors from their own midst is directly related to the degree of danger to themselves that is involved. Another important factor lies in their tendency to downplay the implications of incompetency of their own kind. With their continual need to demonstrate independence and to ward off real (and imagined) threats to autonomy, they are highly sensitized to implications of incompetence that might reflect back on themselves. They are familiar with the popular stereotypes about aging, and, while denying them, they chronically fear the attenuation of their own mental functioning.

In general, the SRO hotel is very permissive of the extremes of human conduct; the economic dependency of such hotels renders them tolerant of behavior that would not be permitted in more respectable hotels.[7] The manager of the Guinevere is ruefully aware of this fact, and he refers to the seventh floor as the "psycho ward," where he puts his "loud nuts." The following episode is an example of the great permissiveness of the SRO slum hotel:

Leo, a veteran, had just been released from Cascade State Mental Hospital. He was living in the hotel. One morning the maid discovered him, sitting in front of his open door, masturbating. Several people complained to the manager. When the maid attempted to clean the

7. In fact, Shapiro, "Reciprocal Dependence," concludes that a primary function of SROs is to perpetuate pathological behavioral patterns by maintaining an ill population in the community.

room, he showed her a gun which he said he was going to use to kill Lorraine [his girl friend], because she had "wired his mind." Then he said that he was going to kill everyone in the hotel and everyone in the universe. The maid called the manager, who called the police. When Leo came down into the lobby later that day, the manager and the police officers attempted to prevent him from leaving the hotel. He began waving the gun around and issuing threats. The police subdued him, and in the process confirmed that his gun was loaded. They handcuffed him and took him away. The manager asked them to be gentle with him. Two months later, the manager let him back into the hotel.

As pointed out before, the manager is more lenient toward the elderly tenants and often tolerates behavior from an elderly permanent that he would not allow a transient. Examples range from incontinence to running battles over the rent. The general pattern of greater latitude that SRO managers allow their elderly long-term residents probably accounts to a significant degree for the continued ability of many of these people with manifest mental and physical disabilities to maintain themselves outside of institutions. Few children, however loving and dutiful, will put up with aging parents who regularly soil their bedclothes and washbasins with feces; few relatives would preserve equanimity in the face of spectacles for which the SRO hotel lobby is often the setting. There is not so much exaggeration as truth to the popular belief that hotel living constitutes a kind of moral holiday.

The activities of Mr. Jones, a sixty-six-year-old former Marine, for example, would not be tolerated in many settings; in the SRO hotel, they hardly produce a raised eyebrow.

> The tenants told me that he is a "procurer" and when I asked them what they meant, thinking they meant that he dealt in stolen goods, they said, "Women, anything he can get." They said, "You see him around here with the fifty-cent variety. He goes down to the bus

depot and picks up young girls who can't find jobs. He persuades them to stay with him; then, he teaches them the ropes, how to shoplift, hook, anything." I was a bit skeptical, especially after talking to Mr. Jones, who was nearly incoherent, talking wildly about first one thing, then the other. He said that he was the karate champion of the world, the most decorated Marine in World War II, an agent for the FBI, a buddy of the head of the Mafia, etc. He contradicted himself several times, and struck me as being about as schizoid as one person possibly could be. I was doubtful that he could get it together enough to run a white slave trade. I was wrong. At least three girls—all young and pretty—served an apprenticeship with him while I was conducting this research. I was able to talk with two of them, and they said that he was really a "nice" man, and not at all like the other "weirdos" down here. The manager said that he had to clamp down on Mr. Jones's operation, as he was going across the border, getting young girls, and bringing them back to the hotel, and the manager feared there would be trouble.

The point that bears reemphasis in understanding the modes of adjustment of these aged SRO tenants is the powerful role played by pervasive deviance. They must contend on a daily basis with threats to their capacity to maintain even minimal survival requirements. This reality renders all aspects of their life style to some degree problematic. The coping skills which they rely upon are shaped by the ubiquitousness of unpredictable events that may victimize them at any time. Additionally, coping skills reflect the disproportionate expenditure of resources required of these people.

The constant drain on inadequate resources leaves little to allocate to fulfilling the so-called higher needs. The development of skills to effect ego enhancement is rudimentary and neglected. Self-actualizing behaviors are a luxury these old people can rarely afford. They are not interested in cultural events: some of the men may attend a nearby pornographic film, and pornographic paperbacks pass from hand to hand, but for the most part the only reading done is the racing sheet in the city newspaper.

The aged tenants of this hotel are discredited people in the eyes of the larger society; to the extent that they are socially visible at all, they are losers. They respond to this image by asserting that outsiders cannot know that there is a great variation in their midst.[8] While some slum hotels may attract disreputable "types," the permanent guests of *their* hotel are a "better class." In line with this, most tenants prefer to associate with residents of other hotels only if they consider them to be on the same level as the Guinevere.

There is a considerable amount of face-saving going on in this group of people. The management of impressions and the establishment of an acceptable social identity takes three principal forms: making comparisons between the Guinevere tenants and the tenants of other SRO hotels in the neighborhood, who are said to be of a "lower class" and are avoided; manufacturing a personal biography that enhances the author; and self-defining to prove oneself superior to the other residents of the Guinevere, a person who really does not "belong here."[9] The following statement by an elderly man, who actively manages the impression he makes on others, gives a picture of how some of these people are able to work out a favorable social identity:

> I have to say that I'm out of it. Yes, I'm not entangled in all the petty associations that people here are con-

8. Shapiro, ibid., portrays SROs as semiclosed social systems which both self-isolate and are isolated from the surrounding community. Contact with the "outside" that occurs is often negative because of the concentration of social and physical pathology, which leads to SROs becoming conspicuous in their neighborhoods through frequent police and ambulance calls, night fights, and stoop loitering.

9. "Each deviant . . . works to neutralize his own deviance and at the same time establishes the deviant character of the other. This procedure is not peculiar to persons in deviant situations. Normal persons also 'rationalize' their morally questionable behavior, often establishing their respectability with reference to someone who is 'really deviant.' The reader is urged to appreciate the universality of the above process." Jacobs, ed., *Getting By*, pp. 64-65.

cerned with. It's just trivial and I really can't be bothered. That's what I mean, I'm out of it. Oh, well, yes, there are some others here, a few like me, who don't belong, if you know what I mean. For instance, Mr. West, he doesn't belong here. I mean, he's superior to those others. But, things happen and here we are. But I try to stay out of it. I can't be bothered.

Impression management and the maintenance of an acceptable social identity are tasks that require specifically interpersonal skills. The aged tenants in the Guinevere attempt, as do all people in all societies, to satisfy self-needs by developing strategies to enhance a self-identity that is favorable to the individual and acceptable to others. They differ only in that they can spare extremely limited resources for this task, and that they can command a much diminished basis of interpersonal support.

CHAPTER FIVE

"Making It"

Truly, "It is a full-time job to be old and poor."[1] That these people are managing to retain their independence is no mean feat, when we consider their multiple physical and mental handicaps and disabilities, their meager economic resources, their lack of access to community services, their own internally atomistic pattern of social relationships. Such marginal patterns of living necessitate a disproportionate expenditure of energy and effort merely to get by, "to make it."

Making it is a constant preoccupation and a major goal for these elderly tenants; in order to accomplish this goal, they use several unconventional ways of supplementing their limited incomes. The Guinevere tenants refer to these unconventional ways of earning a living as hustling, and some sort of hustle constitutes the principal means of making it for most of them. Thus, to hustle is to make it, to engage in some kind of activity —legal or illegal, alone or with a partner—which brings in money to enable the individual to get by. Hustling includes a variety of work situations which, although operated on a stand-

1. Quoted from Curtin, *Nobody Ever Died of Old Age,* p. 56. Research into the occupational activities of elderly SRO tenants is urgently needed, as a shortcoming of previous studies lies in their almost total neglect of this issue. Members of the hotel society generate and sustain characteristic ways of making a living and providing for economic necessities. Unfortunately, we know very little about these matters.

by and unstable basis, and capable at best of generating only sporadic and minimal funds, nevertheless allows these elderly hotel occupants to take care of their basic needs and maintain independent living arrangements.

The term "hustling" is a familiar one in the lexicons of many minority and subcultural groups in American society. It is a term indicative of the harsh realities of marginal status in the social structure of conventional society. It refers to some kind of effort that is aimed at obtaining desired ends, regardless of conventional ethics; often the hustle involves some risk, and by definition hustles are not stable kinds of work situations. They are operated on an ad hoc basis, and must adapt to the fluctuating conditions that characterize many forms of marginal living. Hustling differs from conventional work situations in that it lacks legitimacy and social approval and support; it confers no approved status within conventional society; and it is not a dependable source of income. The hustle work situation demands that the individual continually seek to manipulate and structure situations so as to serve his immediate interests. The extremely problematic character of hustling is demonstrated in this definition elicited from an elderly Guinevere tenant, who "hawks" balloons on the street: " . . . a way of working for people who can't get any steady employment. A guy does it because he's got no other thing to fall back on. He can't get no other job, no secure job. He does it 'cause he's got to, and he don't make no real money. He just gets by."

The elderly tenants in the Guinevere live in poverty; the majority are receiving public assistance. The monthly or bi-weekly check is insufficient for many of them, and they must find ways to supplement their incomes. They must, in short, find work.[2] However, there are strong deterrents to this. Dis-

2. The gerontological literature is replete with general studies of the fate of the older worker, the semiretired older worker, and the retired older worker. See Carp's study of the occupational characteristics of the aged slum dweller, for whom retirement—usually from menial jobs that provided no security, tenure, or fringe benefits—has not been an event that occurred on a given day, but was rather the culmination of increasingly frequent and

criminative hiring practices with regard to the over-fifty worker are common enough throughout society. Many of these people have few or obsolete work skills. Additionally, poor health and mental and physical disabilities render some of them virtually unemployable. In the competitive sphere of job situations, these people are at the bottom of the heap. Many have poor work records and probably could not handle a steady job. Among them are heavy drinkers and chronic alcoholics who have histories of irregular work habits that have gradually eliminated employment opportunities for them.

A small number have found more or less steady conventional jobs in low-paying, low-skill services, working as waiters, dishwashers, cleanup helpers. Even these jobs, with their abysmally low pay scales, little security, and poor working conditions, are

---

lengthy periods of time during which these individuals were unable to obtain employment. Carp, "The Mobility of Older Slum-dwellers."

Several studies have found that the loss of the occupational role marks a dramatic turning point in the lives of the elderly. Preston, in a study of retired and nonretired aged, found that the retired group experienced more role confusion, shared the invidious stereotypes of older people which prevail in American culture, and were greatly lacking in confidence as to the possibility of their being included in meaningful social activities. Preston, "Traits Endorsed by Older Non-retired and Retired Subjects." Carp, in a study which included elderly persons who worked for pay, did volunteer work, or did not work at all, concluded that those who worked for pay more frequently identified themselves as middle-aged and were more likely to perceive themselves as useful and important. Carp, "Differences Among Older Workers, Volunteers, and Persons Who Are Neither." Meltzer found that the closer an individual gets to retirement, the more ambivalent he feels about his future status. With the advent of actual retirement, the individual is likely to perceive his role as unproductive and his status as not socially legitimized. Meltzer, "Age Differences in Happiness and Life Adjustments of Workers." Miller points out that the occupational identity of the individual establishes his position in the social system, allowing others to evaluate his status and role, and providing a context within which his social activity can be interpreted. On the other hand, the retired individual "finds himself without a functional role which would justify his social future and without an identity which would provide a concept of self which is tolerable to him and acceptable to others." Miller, "The Social Dilemma of the Aging Leisure Participant." The overall conclusions of many of these studies is that the giving up of the work role and the assuming of a leisure role involves nearly traumatic consequences for many elderly individuals. In some perverse fashion, the necessity for the Guinevere tenants to continue to work aids in their continued ability to function psychologically (as well as economically).

at a premium in the area. Most of these aged people cannot get conventional jobs; for them, the hustle is the only feasible alternative.[3]

The Guinevere tenants distinguish nine common types of hustling activity: (1) "conning," (2) "go-fors," (3) shoplifting, (4) scavenging, (5) "pushers," (6) prostitution (male and female), (7) "dingman," (8) begging or panhandling, and (9) peddling. Each kind of hustle involves an exchange of goods (with the possible exception of begging), requires the mastery of job-related skills, such as special argots, and in a minimal way permits the individual to realize the all-important goal of making it.

"Conning" has both general and specific meanings. The broad meaning is that the con is a strategy used to obtain some desired end by employing a verbal deception. Thus, the ruse to forestall the management from plugging one's room, and the manufactured life history to enhance social identity, are common uses of the con. In this sense, conning is a ubiquitous activity that serves a variety of personal aims in a number of different situations. In the more specific sense of the term, the con is a hustle designed to procure material goods. Then the con is most often employed in conjunction with another hustle. Examples would include the conning which the peddler does in persuading a prospective customer of the quality of his merchandise; the "poor me" story that the prostitute uses to garner a larger profit from her client; the efforts that the shoplifter makes to convince his customer of the legality of a particular item. The higher the degree of verbal skill—that is, the better the "con job"—the more successful the individual will be at gaining his desired end. There is considerable competition

3. It should be stressed that I have defined hustling *not* in terms of external criteria—that is, not by referring to the sociological literature—but rather in terms of the definitions utilized by the tenants. For a discussion of the strategy of "grounding" concepts through the data-collection stage of a research project, the reader is referred to several works by Glaser and Strauss, namely, *The Discovery of Grounded Theory*; "Discovery of Grounded Theory"; and "Discovery of Substantive Theory."

among them as to who can con better, and "telling a good story" confers prestige. Conning is a strategy used for the most part to obtain something from "outsiders" (prospective customers) or from the hotel staff. However, attempts to con each other are not uncommon.[4]

"Go-fors" or "runners" are individuals who engage in a certain kind of activity for money or alcohol. For a small amount of change—a dime, a quarter, rarely more—they go for small items, such as cigarettes, coffee, foodstuffs, wine. Many of the individuals who hustle in this fashion are chronic alcoholics who use the money earned to keep themselves supplied with liquor. In some cases, part of the agreement will be a share in the bottle brought back to the customer.

A number of the tenants practice shoplifting for the express purpose of selling the "hot items." Shoplifting for items that the individual plans to keep for himself is not considered a hustle. The hustle involves selling the goods to someone else. Items such as clothing, jewelry, and small appliances top the list. Buyers are usually other tenants in the Guinevere, or tenants in nearby SROs. The profession is not well developed and brings only a small return to those individuals in the hotel who do it. There is only one more venturesome and professional individual who shoplifts "on order" for specific items for buyers and also disposes of some items through a "fence."

Scavenging is a hustle in which the individual collects junk from trash cans and then carts his finds off to one of the "we buy anything" stores. Although the tenants know of such activities and know tenants at other hotels who do it, they insist that no one at the Guinevere has to resort to this way of earning a living. In fact, there are a small number of tenants in the hotel who sporadically collect and sell castoff items to supplement their finances. Scavenging is a low-status hustle, and less common than the other unconventional work situations discussed thus far.

4. The reader is, no doubt, wondering if attempts to con and manipulate me were common. In answer, I might ask, "Is Los Angeles in California?"

By "pushers" they mean individuals who sell narcotics illegally. They agree that "pushing" is a young person's hustle, and tend to link it with the "transients" and blacks in the area. The sentiment is usually expressed that elderly people are not interested or involved in the illegal market for drugs. There is a small market for certain painkillers and soporific drugs, however, and occasionally one of the elderly tenants might practice a hustle involving drugs.

Prostitution is a familiar hustle; the neighborhood abounds with "hookers" of both sexes. Some of the men may find themselves the victims of this hustle, for often enough a related hustle is the "rolling" of the client by the prostitute's "agent" (pimp). The elderly men are vulnerable to intimidation and force, and represent an easy "mark." It is interesting that the oldest profession can find a place in its ranks for some of the aged women in the hotel, who cannot find a place in the conventional job market. There are two elderly women living in the Guinevere who occasionally "turn tricks" to pay their rent. There are other instances of activities geared toward an exchange of goods, which are borderline and could be broadly defined as prostitution. For example, there is an elderly barmaid who goes out with the men and exchanges her sexual favors for what she calls her "tip money."

The "dingman" is an individual who sells Veterans of Foreign Wars pins and paper flowers to unsuspecting customers, who are led to believe that the profits go to charity. In fact, they are for the seller. The dingman may strengthen his appeal by wearing an old army outfit; he may con his customers by pleading with them to "give something for the boys." He may refer to his war wound. This hustle is practiced by both young and old tenants in the hotel and is exclusively a male hustle.

Begging or panhandling is a low-status hustle; it is something that *other* people at *other* hotels do. It is similar to scavenging in this regard, for none of the tenants openly admits to panhandling. (There is one notable exception. An elderly man in the Guinevere travels all over the country begging. He has lived in the hotel for a number of years and is regarded by the other tenants as a "real character." Since he has "style," the tenants define his begging as an activity above common panhandling.)

By far the most common hustle is peddling. Over a third of the elderly men in the hotel peddle more or less regularly to supplement their income. Various terms are used in referring to these individuals—peddlers, hawkers, hustlers, carnies. Reflective of the prevalence of peddling as the dominant type of hustling activity, the term "hustler" is often used synonymously with "peddler." They are also called "carnies," and many of them speak "carnese" or "carny talk," a mixture of pig latin and underworld slang spoken by the peddlers with prior connections with carnivals and circuses. The peddlers are dependent upon each other to realize economic gain; a person can peddle alone, but it is more efficient and profitable to establish working relationships. The work relationships established by the carnies display a stability not seen otherwise in the Guinevere society, and, indeed, these hustlers constitute the most identifiable and durable social grouping in the hotel. Also, as a group they enjoy the respect (and frequently envy) of the other tenants. It is one of those ironies of SRO life that these men who hawk balloons and plastic pennants through the city streets are engaging in what their social world considers to be a high-status hustle.

TOP DOGS AND UNDERDOGS

There exists a status hierarchy among these individuals that ranks hustles (and hustlers). The criteria for determining which hustles are high or low status are: (1) the more economically profitable, the higher the status of a specific hustle; (2) the greater the regularity and dependability of the hustle, the higher the status; and (3) the more individual autonomy afforded by a specific hustle, the higher the status.

Conversely, the less secure the hustle, the smaller the remuneration, the lower the status of the hustle and hustler. Exemplified in "go-fors," scavenging, and panhandling, such low-status hustles are avoided by the more resourceful individuals. Thus, the alcoholic "go-for," whose payoff entails only a swig from the client's bottle, is generally considered to be a fool.

The avoidance of dependency has a significant impact on the nature of the hustle employed, as evidenced by the fact that many hustlers operate as loners and are suspicious of shared endeavors. This preference for single-person hustles, or at most hustles which require a minimum of partners, is a pattern that embodies several of the dominant norms of SRO society—independence, suspicion, and the manipulation of others to serve one's personal ends. Indeed, the latter is particularly revealing in its relation to status differences among hustlers. The carnies, in particular, are seen as the personification of the independent loners who make it, neither asking for quarter nor giving it, in the harsh world of the SRO. The panhandler, on the other hand, arouses contempt because of his subordinate position vis-à-vis his customer. Thus, the embodiment of the major SRO norms is a significant standard by which tenants rank hustling situations and each other as hustlers.

Certain job-related skills—such as amount of training necessary to master the hustle, the use of a special argot, and relative importance of "connections"—also figure in distinguishing between hustles. Some hustles require that the novice serve a kind of informal apprenticeship under someone more experienced, whereas other hustles can be done by almost anyone with little or no training. Those hustles that require a more formalized training period include peddling and shoplifting; "go-fors" and panhandlers, on the other hand, require almost no preparation or skill.

Another job-related skill is the mastery of a special argot. The carny talk of the street peddlers is the prototype, and other argots developed and used by individuals in specific hustle work situations are basically spin-offs from this colorful language derived from the carnival world. Further, mastery of carnese is indicative of the separation hustlers insist upon maintaining between themselves and "outsiders," that is, nonhustlers.

The importance of connections to the performance of the hustle varies greatly. The network of individuals involved in the carnie's business enterprise is (by SRO standards) dense. From the "backer" who "fronts" him money to buy stock, to the carny "boss," to the friendly merchant who charges only a nominal sum for the use of the "privilege," the carny uses a number of individuals to insure the success of his hustle. The beggar, however, works alone and can rely on no one to facilitate his hustle.

A final distinction between hustle situations involves the complexity of relationships and roles necessary to sustain different hustles. Hustle situations vary in the degree to which they are characteristically single-person endeavors or multiple-person operations. Those hustles that require more than a single individual working alone, typically require a clear-cut division of labor, with role rights and obligations. Thus, "dingman," "go-fors," and panhandlers are carried out by individuals working alone. Shoplifting, as practiced in the Guinevere, is typically a single-person hustle. Prostitution and street peddling are usually multiple-person hustles. The carnies, whose hustle is more often a multiple-person endeavor, are able to maintain their favored status because their dependency upon others is confined to other carnies and does not extend beyond the economic contingencies of peddling. Of course, the fundamental reason for their high status rests upon the overall higher economic gain in their enterprise.[5]

5. This chapter is adapted from "On Being Excluded: An Analysis of Elderly and Adolescent Street Hustlers," by Clifford English and Joyce Stephens, and is reprinted from *Urban Life and Culture*, vol. 4, no. 2 (July 1975), by permission of the publisher, Sage Publications, Inc.

CHAPTER SIX

Carnies and Marks

Their place of business is the street corner, the ball park, the fairground, in short, any place where public and civic events are taking place. There is a specialization among the carnies determined on the basis of the type of merchandise they are selling. There are flower hustlers, food hustlers (hot dogs, beverages, and the like), novelty hustlers (balloons, pennants, dolls), and all-around hustlers (who switch around and do not sell only one kind of item). The tendency is to specialize in a particular kind of merchandise.

Hustlers are dependent upon each other to realize economic gain. One person can peddle alone, but it is more efficient and profitable to establish working partnerships, and this pattern is the common one. These work relationships display a stability not seen otherwise in the world of the Guinevere aged. In this society of severely attenuated relationships and impoverished social roles, the carnies are nearly unique. The primary source of cohesion is the exigencies that arise in the course of arranging the hustle, with secondary sources being generated from the common experiences, interests, and frequently backgrounds peculiar to their hustle. The solidarity that one finds among the carnies is strengthened by their recognition of the necessity for mutual cooperation for economic gain, and tends to resemble the other relational bonds formed in this hotel society—that is, tends to be instrumental and nonintimate.

In terms of the norms of the larger society, hawking and peddling cheap merchandise through the city streets and selling hot dogs at ball games or balloons at carnivals are not usually considered prestige-conferring occupations. But at the Guinevere, the carnies are viewed with both admiration and respect. In their independent and aggressive stance, they have come to typify one of the major values of these people—the denial and defeat of dependency. The carnies are defined and self-defined as a special breed. Even those few individuals at the Guinevere who have sufficient financial assets to live comfortably do not enjoy the respect or status that the carnies do.

The most significant factor in the carnies' work situation is the hustle. They spend countless hours seeking it out, arranging their time and energies around it, defining and establishing relationships in terms of it. The carnies usually work in twos and threes; this structuring of the work situation into partnerships is characterized by differentiated roles. The roles articulated are the "boss" and his workers. The boss assumes the major burden of responsibility for setting up the hustle. He must purchase the stock, take care of it until it is to be sold, select the event, arrange for transportation to the event, arrange for and pay for the "privilege," and supervise the day's work activity. The boss is the one who makes all of the major decisions, including the hiring of workers to sell merchandise up and down the streets.

Carrying most of the responsibility for the success of the hustle, the boss is likely to be a skilled peddler himself. The traits which most distinguish these men who assume leadership roles in the hustling trade are: prior experience with peddling (carnivals, circuses, concession stands); marked organizational skills; certain job-related skills that are specifically geared to the hustle, such as "conning" ability; ownership or access to a car; mastery of carnese; and the right "connections."

The boss hires other men to peddle his merchandise on the street while he remains at the "privilege" with the bulk of the merchandise and sells from this location. Some bosses set up temporary flimsy stalls, others work out of their cars. The privilege is not free, and costs range from ten to twenty dollars a day. The privilege may be in front of a gas station or perhaps the corner of a parking lot; the owner of the business sets a price, and the carny boss either meets it or moves on in search of a more reasonable privilege. Rarely, a carny who has worked an event for years may be able to get his privilege free from a friendly merchant. The privilege is considered to be a crucial factor in the success of the hustle, and locations as close to the attraction as possible are at a premium. Much rivalry develops among the carny bosses over who will get the best privilege, and the bosses are judged by other carnies on the basis of their ability to arrange for a good privilege. [1]

The working partnership of the boss and his workers is not democratic. The boss makes the decisions and also accepts most of the responsibility for the hustle. The boss determines the rate of pay—usually a flat amount (twenty dollars for a day's work is an average)—or, in some cases, a percentage of the take. Better hawkers will bargain for higher pay, but it is the boss who decides. The workers, for their part, are required to do basically one thing—sell the merchandise where the boss tells them to. Typically, this will be up and down the street, covering the location of the greatest activity and the largest concentration of people. A cardinal violation of the working agreement occurs when a worker "leaves the street," that is, stops selling while there is still merchandise. Bosses evaluate their workers primarily on their dependability, which is defined in terms of willingness to walk and hawk goods all day and all night, or as long as the stock holds out. If the boss feels that they have done well enough to take a breather, he will signal his workers, but it is not their place to make this decision.

Workers prefer to work with certain bosses and not with others. The criteria they use to judge a good boss are: he locates good events, arranges to have sufficient stock, gets a good privi-

---

1. A list of carny terms begins on p. 111.

lege, displays his stock well, keeps an eye on the money, and pays his workers according to a prearranged scale. These working partnerships shift membership frequently, as fallings-out occur between bosses and workers due to disagreements over pay, professional rivalry, bosses who have insufficient stock, workers who get drunk and "leave the streets."

A typical work day begins early, six or seven o'clock in the morning. The boss—having selected an event that he thinks will draw a large crowd, purchased stock from a wholesaler in novelties, and hired as many workers as he thinks he will need —arrives with his workers at the privilege and sets up for the day. They try to arrange the stock in ways that will catch the attention of passers-by. "Flash" (showy merchandise) is displayed prominently.

Balloons are blown up, mechanical toys are wound up, and the workers start walking the streets. The day will be a long one; they will not leave until very late at night. While the stock holds out, the weather is tolerable, and the customers keep coming, they will continue to cry their wares and add their own hues to the street colors.

The boss's control over the operation can be seen in his relationship to his workers. Not only does he assign the work, but he maintains control over the money. The workers wear aprons with pockets or carry small pouches known as "grouch bags" in which they deposit the money and make change. Each time they sell out, they return to the boss for more stock, and they are required to hand over the money they have collected. The boss keeps all of the proceeds except change money. Thus, he controls the money and makes sure that there is no pilfering. Indeed, the boss is the only one who knows how much money they are pulling in during the day. The workers never object to or question this strategy; they expect the boss to be responsible for the money.

Reinforcing this system of mutual definitions as to appropriate work roles is the expectation that the boss will shoulder the primary responsibility for realizing a major goal of the hustling work situation: he must "cover the stock," that is, earn enough money to pay for the investment in stock. Anything above this amount is profit. The boss is responsible for determining that the stock has been covered, and to this end he counts the money several times during the day, hoping to reach the sum that equalizes his expenditure. Once this occurs, there is a discernible change of pace. The boss becomes more talkative; he pushes his workers less; and, in general, a more relaxed atmosphere develops. The workers recognize these cues and may begin to slack off. The pace becomes less strenuous, and rests more frequent and longer in duration. Now they will probably eat lunch, and the boss may send one of his workers to buy a bottle to pass around. Other hustlers from different work groups may drop by to chat and complain about what a terrible day it has been for them and to swap stories of how it used to be in the good old days. Yet they know how long to stay and when to take their leave, as this territory has been paid for, and they will return to their own privilege to do any selling.

In the course of a work day, the carnies come into contact with several groups who may stand in important relationships to them and their economic endeavors. These groups include other hustlers, customers, and people who may be in a position either to facilitate or to hinder the hustler's operation.

The relationships between rival hustlers is of particular interest. There is considerable professional jealousy and a fierce spirit of competition among them. Carnies continually compare their own skill, experience, and savvy with the shortcomings of other hustlers. There is agreement that some hustlers are better than others, the best hustler being defined as the one who sells the most stock and makes the greatest profit. The most compelling criterion of success in their profession is economic gain. Accompanying the jealousy are attitudes of suspicion and distrust aroused by other hustlers who "ask too many questions" or stray onto another's privilege for too long. Carnies will "dummy up" and become very secretive if they suspect that another hustler is trying to hustle them. The strongly competitive cast of the hustling trade is understandable when viewed in the context of marginal and unreliable profits; at best, there is a limited market for the goods, and there are certainly enough risks and pitfalls in this occupation to render its success a constant question.

Contacts between the carny and his customers are suffused with a barely concealed hostility and distrust, particularly from the perspective of the peddler. Carnies are well aware of the low repute in which they are held by "outsiders." The term "outsider" refers to anyone who is not a member of the carny subculture, and also, broadly, to conventional society. Other terms are "mark" and "sucker," which reflect the attitudes of contempt and hostility of the carny toward persons and groups outside his occupation. A basic consensus underlies the reactions of carnies to this conflict; they reject the definitions of conventional society, which entail negative conceptions of both the peddler and peddling. Reinforcing each other, the carnies are able by prolonged interaction to generate counter definitions which stress the legitimacy and worthiness of their occupation and its practitioners.

Carnies respond to the negative judgments of conventional society in two fundamental ways: by the belief in a carny "mystique" that provides an alternate set of self-definitions, and by a deliberate strategy of self-segregation and isolation from the norms and standards of conventional society. These patterns are self-reinforcing and permit the carny to maintain a favorable view of self, to define broadly what kinds of activities are considered proper, and to disregard generally the standards of conventional society.

The carny "mystique" is related to the fact that most carnies' full-time activity centers around hustling, and consequently, the self is deeply involved in this occupation. Carnies assert that they are a "special breed"—independent, individualistic, tough, and "in the know." Further, the mystique posits them as possessing skills that set them apart from nonhustlers. This attitude is generalized into a feeling that carnies are different from and better than other kinds of people. They enjoy a special talent for sizing up people and seeing behind their respectable fronts. The development of an alternate and acceptable conception of self and one's activities is a consequence of the conflict that carnies feel to be inherent in their relation to outsiders. This feeling of being a different kind of person who leads a different kind of life is deep-seated and continually reinforced by the carnies in their interaction with each other.[2]

Supporting carny definitions of self and occupation as worthy and legitimate (if misunderstood by others) is a process of deliberate self-segregation and isolation. The carnies prefer their own kind and associate almost exclusively with other peddlers both on and off the job. Their use of carnese is further evidence of the process of self-segregation. Mastery of carny talk identifies another hustler, whereas the lack of it or improper usage immediately reveals the outsider. The interests and concerns of this group emphasize their isolation from nonhustlers. While some of this segregation is a consequence of the conditions of the work situation, much of it develops out of the carnies' hostility and distrust of outsiders. The carnies derive much satisfaction from "putting down" clients, and often regale each other with tales attesting to the stupidity and greed of their "marks." The carny prefers to limit his interaction with outsiders to those situations, manipulated by the carny, in which he (the carny) can obtain from the client the money so desired. Of course, as the mystique claims, against the experienced carny, the "mark" does not stand a chance.

The customer (outsider) is a necessary ingredient in the carny's occupation, though, for it is his money that the hustler is after. To achieve this separation of the customer from his mon-

2. I acknowledge my indebtedness to Howard S. Becker's analysis of the dance musician for some of the central ideas in this discussion of the carnies' handling of nonhustlers. See Becker, *Outsiders,* chap. 5, "The Culture of a Deviant Group: The Dance Musician," and chap. 6, "Careers in a Deviant Occupational Group: The Dance Musician."

ey, the hustler skillfully manages impressions: he is the funny balloon man to the children; he is not above appealing to their sympathy; many times he is as colorful and entertaining as the event they came to see. To the hustler, the customer is primarily the "mark," the "sucker" who will buy the "junk." In the words of one hustler: "Can you believe the junk these marks will buy? Those rubbers [balloons] are low-line [cheap] and a nickel would be more than they're worth. But the suckers'll pay a quarter for'em, so that's all right with me."

There are some people whom the carny does not want hanging around his privilege. Children without money are run off and told not to come back unless they get some money from their parents. Rowdies can be a problem, as joking escalates into roughhousing. Selling on the streets is vulnerable physically as well as socially and economically, and the hustler is well aware of the potential dangers to himself and his enterprise. To lessen the risk of being robbed, the hustler curries favor with attending police officers. He makes it a practice to strike up conversations with officers as they pass by his stall, and gives them "a little something to take home for the kids." In return, the officers keep an eye out for the safety of the hustler, thus affording at least some element of protection should an emergency arise.

Other individuals who frequently are in a position to influence the hustlers' work situation include merchants and owners of stores located close to the event. They may take advantage of the situation by asking very high amounts for a good privilege; or, conversely, as a favor to an old man, they may charge only a nominal sum. Worst of all, they may run off the peddlers and threaten to call the police if they come back.

There is the usual assortment of gatekeeper types at any event. Their duties include checking to see if the hustlers have their peddlers' licenses (three dollars per year) and, in many instances, making sure that the peddlers do not intrude beyond a certain defined area. For example, at one of the parades that I attended with many of the carnies from the Guinevere, the vendors were not allowed to sell inside a large park where people had gathered to watch fireworks. They could work outside the park, on the streets, and up to the park entrance, but not inside. Such exclusion makes the street vendors very angry.

The contingencies of the hustling trade that may spell the difference between success and failure are many. Bad weather can be disastrous. The boss is not always sure that the event he has selected will draw a large and free-spending crowd. The carnies maintain that some neighborhoods are better than others. Certainly, a poorly located privilege can mean a ruinous day. The stock may not appeal and be difficult to push. Or it may include too many "larrys," that is, defective merchandise, which will reduce the profit. Insufficient stock means a loss, too. Winter is a lean time for the carnies; more events are held indoors, and exclusionary policies and quotas increase the competition.

The marginality of hustling bears repeated emphasis. On a bad day the hustler will not make enough to cover his stock; he will not be able to pay his workers; he will have to store his stock until another event; he will not meet his debts; nobody will be happy. On a good day, with sufficient stock, he may double his money. For example, when "Aristotle," a carny boss, worked novelties on the Fourth of July with two workers, they had a good day. He had invested $125.00 in stock, and he took in $307.00 that day. His expenses included the stock, $12.00 for the privilege, $30.00 apiece for his two workers, lunch and dinner for himself and his workers, and two bottles of gin. His personal profit was about $100.00. What must be borne in mind is the irregular nature of this work: a hustler may work as often as two or three times a week and as infrequently as once a month or less. Thus, hustling as practiced by the carnies is not a steady source of income. Hustling is replete with multiple uncertainties, and, in addition, there are long intervals when there is no hustle.

There is a pride of workmanship among the carnies; they insist that they are different from the other elderly residents in the Guinevere, who do not hustle on the streets for a living. Their work situation and the group of colleagues that develops around it contribute to their own sense of social identity:

> I've worked rubbers and pennants for years. Worked the state fair for years. Used to go to fairs in Georgia, Florida, all over, selling. Worked for Ringling Brothers Circus for twenty-seven years. But I can't go now, too crippled up for all that driving. I go to the fair and the sports events and parades on holidays here in the city and suburbs. Oh, I might get as far as Greystown for something big. Trouble is, you can't always tell if it's gonna be worth it. I get a list and decide which ones to buy stock for, oh, like the state fair, that's always when I can plan to sell a lotta stock. And the parades in Los Ellos: those are good people. They spend a lotta money; they take care of their children. They come out for parades; they're good family people. I like that community. People don't know, they think anybody can be a vendor. Why, I broke in Butch over there, and look at him, his pennants draggin' the ground. He doesn't know how to sell properly. Doesn't even know how to display his stock so people can see it and want to buy it. He'll never be a good seller. This kind of work isn't for everybody. The hours are killing. It's more cut out for a person who is rugged. I'm an old man; I'm crippled up, but I need something to do. I'm not goin' to give up, why, look at some of the old people here, right in the lobby. They're just waitin' to die, a lot of 'em. But I go right out selling; I've got to be where I can do something. We carnies are tough, you know what I'm tryin' to say.

Carnese borrows heavily from the argot of carnival people and various sectors of the underworld. It is as colorful and rich in imagery as the nicknames that hustlers assign to each other —for example, Tomato Face, Dutch, The Horse Thief, Dave the Pro, The Rainmaker, Transplant, The Gypsy, Tom the Cool, Back-to-Back Bennie, Louis the Louse, Hot Dog Johnny, The Mad Turk, Crooked Neck Johnson, Hot Stove Louie, Single-Load George, Mother Goose, Big City, Willie the Creep. (The carnies bestowed a nickname on me, "Anywhere," which they explained referred to the fact that I would "fit in anywhere.") Carnese, in common with other argots, is indicative of social bonding and, in the case of the street vendors, grows out of the contingencies of the hustle work situation. Its use is neither accidental nor without purpose; on the contrary, it serves the specific function of indicating that an outsider is within earshot. Thus, one hustler may advise another hustler to "dummy up," there's a "herring in the place," which means, "keep quiet, there's a suspicious-looking person asking questions."

The carnies utilize this argot to regulate interaction with outsiders and to preserve their trade secrets. Thus, the adoption of carnese reflects their attitudes and the norms which define the relationships of hustlers to nonhustlers. Their relationships to outsiders are always established and structured in terms of the hustle and the kinds of transactions that will facilitate it. These transactions are based on the definition of the outsider as one who will either help or hinder the proposed hustle. The outsider is always someone to be sold, to be conned, to be hustled—the outsider is a potential customer. The image of the customer as foolish runs through the argot of the hustlers, and many carny stories are geared toward revealing how gullible people are conned into paying through the nose by smooth-talking hustling men. The use of a special argot is another instance of the hustlers' self-defining based upon common work experiences and necessities, an attempt to maintain boundaries that divide them and the hustling experience from others and sustain their identity as a distinct social group.

CHAPTER SEVEN

Men and Women

The world of the Guinevere aged is a society composed largely of men, and in this way it is typical of SRO hotel populations. Elderly women are considerably less likely to wind up in slum hotels; they tend to live with family members or in their own homes or apartments. The few women who do live in the hotel are in significant ways differentiated from the men.

The dominant values of the SRO society come into conflict with the values supporting sex-role identities in the case of the women. For them, the consequences include a reduced capacity to cope, a greater vulnerability, and an even more extreme isolation and loneliness than the men endure. Particularly, they are deficient in the all-important value of independence. The tenants recognize and often remark on the subversion of this major value:

> It don't matter how old a woman gets. They're always clingy, just hopin' to depend on some man.

> They want others to cater to them, to fawn on them. They try to be dependent, but the men won't put up with it. So, they're more helpless and foolish and lonelier, too, desperately lonely.

> The men are in better shape mentally. I mean, because they're independent and have practicality. But

these women are looking for someone to lean on. The men get by, they manage, like, take the "carnies." They get out and around. They don't stay in the hotel, they "hustle." But the women aren't like the men—level-headed and practical. Why, they're just like old housewives who can't stick to the point, who expect others to do things for them while they set [*sic*] home. And the men won't have anything to do with them. They know they're just trying to get something out of them.

The theme of "trying to get something out of them" runs through the relationships established between the men and women. The men are wary and suspicious; the women bitter and resentful. Each assumes that the other is trying to use and exploit him (or her).

The probability of these aged men and women working out sustained relationships with each other is attenuated not only by the normative pattern of avoiding intimacy and binding relationships that constitutes both a basal common meaning in their society and a major coping stratagem, but also by conflicting expectancies and demands generated by sex-role prescriptions prevalent in the larger society. The sex-role differences of these people play out the culmination of the conventional culture's sex-role identity assignments.[1]

For the elderly male tenant in the SRO hotel, the taken-for-granted meanings of this society are capable of being synchronized with lifelong male role definitions. For the elderly female tenant, however, sex-role patterns of a lifetime are at odds with the assumptions of SRO life. Therefore, the men experience less role discontinuity, because such dominant values of the SRO environment as decision-making, independence, behaviors emphasizing *instrumentality*, are compatible with the sex-role

1. That the major institutions of American society are permeated with sexist value orientations and discriminatory practices is so obvious that it scarcely bears repeating; nevertheless in this group of elderly persons, the tragic and inevitable consequences are especially prominent. Norman Mailer may be wrong about just about everything else, but he was dead-on when he opined that one pays for everything in life.

identities and demands that they have lived with more or less all their adult lives. For the women, there is a severe break from such traditionally defined sex-role behaviors as nurturing and homemaking, behaviors emphasizing *expressiveness*, that are characterized by their complementary status to the male role.

The elderly women in the Guinevere Hotel have not always lived in slum hotels; they have not always been alone. They, more than the men, are likely to have been married, to have raised children, and to have been linked to the conventional life presented by the larger society. Roles of a lifetime, especially those that play such a crucial part in buttressing selfhood, do not die easily; thus, the elderly women are prone to attempt to retain these role definitions, behaviors, and associated values regarding self and others, and to act in terms of them.[2] Behaviors so inappropriate to the SRO society are countered by sharp rebuff. The men are wary and determined not to be drawn into relationships which they cannot afford, and to this end they define the women as foolish, boring, and a burden if one is silly enough to give them an opening. The men avoid the women and, in so doing, contribute to a deepening sex-related isolation.

The women appear more vulnerable, less successful at coping, unreconciled to their status. A favorite and familiar story of these women tells of the solicitous care still available to them from their families. All they have to do is pick up the telephone and make a call, and the son, daughter, grandchild, whoever, will come for them, take them home, care for them. There is no

2. I might note that the concept of "role" dominates the theoretical frameworks utilized by researchers in the field of aging. There is general agreement that the aged suffer from loss of roles and role-associated relationships. The aged are faced not only with major changes in the cluster of roles that define and integrate them into society, but with the additional trauma of an actual loss of roles. Ernest Burgess refers to the loss of occupational identity and functional roles as a state of being imprisoned in a roleless role. Burgess, ed., *Aging in Western Societies*. However, in the general population of the elderly, role discontinuity is experienced more severely by males; whereas in SRO society, it is the aged woman who suffers more acutely from role loss.

viable basis for these daydreams: children are gone or dead, grandchildren are uninvolved or, in some cases, have actively avoided and refused to have anything to do with these women. Nevertheless, it is a favorite story, even if no one believes it.[3]

The women are less in tune with things; they are not aware of current events, political issues. They, more than the men, try to live in the past or in their reconstructions of imagined pasts, in which they are surrounded by loving families, in which they are "somebody." The adjustment of the women to the world of the SRO is more fragile, more tenuous than that of the men. Ironically, their inappropriate need to revive ways of relating that would allow intimacy is looked upon in the society of SRO tenants as a cover-up for an exploitative ruse, another hustle.

The result is that the women become even more isolated and alone than the men, for the men have relinquished the need for intimacy in order to take care of more basic needs, whose satisfaction precludes all forms of intimacy and dependence. The women are shunned, and efforts on their part to initiate contact are viewed with suspicion. Holdover values from another time—family, children, friendship—are inimical to survival in the world of the SRO. The world of the SRO is a tough, hostile

3. Weakness of kinship ties is, in fact, characteristic of the elderly in America. This pattern is not a recent development; rather, it has roots in the development and expansion of our country. The pattern of European settlement and colonization of North America mitigated against the retention of close kinship ties between the adult generations in the United States. The household size of early America was typically not inclusive of several generations; thus, the extended family was never a dominant pattern in our society. The aged have always been spatially and culturally separated from their adult children and grandchildren. Even where intergenerational ties are maintained, the consequences for both young and old are frequently unsatisfying. Payne notes that continued contact of the aged with their adult children does not necessarily alleviate feelings of uselessness and isolation; indeed, for many elderly people, this is a humbling experience. After a lifetime of making one's own decisions, to be forced outside oneself and one's own age category for information and for value support necessary to make day-to-day decisions, often induces powerfully negative feelings toward oneself and toward one's offspring. Payne, "Some Theoretical Approaches to the Sociology of Aging."

place which phases out the need for intimacy and dependency. For the women, this involves giving up roles and attitudes more sharply and profoundly bound up with their sex identity than is true of the men.

One stratagem for dealing with this conflict which comes to assume a major part in the adjustment of these women is a self-imposed isolation. What begins as enforced isolation merges into a kind of self-isolating as they learn (perforce) to live according to the taken-for-granted meanings that define the reality of the SRO society. That they have not learned as well as the men is occasionally revealed in their conversations which center around past status, prestige, and familial relationships, and in their furtive attempts to make contacts with the men and establish quasi-family relationships. Such lapses are generally met with derision and hostility, so that, over time, these violations of the norms are so carefully guarded against that the women appear to be more unapproachable, independent, and forbidding than the men. But once we get past their chilly exterior, we find vulnerable and unbelievably lonely people. Their management of social identity represents an enforced adaptation in order to make it in the world of the SRO.

The avoidance that characterizes relationships between the sexes does not mean that there is no inter-sex mingling. The men occasionally seek out female company—typically, the services of a prostitute. Next to sports, the horses, and alcohol, sex is the most popular topic of conversation among the men. The hotel is worked by prostitutes from the area and a few part-timers who live in the hotel itself. When the social security checks arrive on the first of the month, the "prossies" arrive also; all ages, often on narcotics, and attended by the ever watchful eye of their "sponsor" (pimp), they pour into the hotel bar to work the old men.[4] Additionally, there are a few middle-

4. Interviews with several police officers and plain-clothes detectives assigned to the area confirmed my observation that little is being done to discourage the trade in bodies. The officers said that they used to pick up the girls for suspicion of being a disorderly person, but the courts ruled that they

aged and elderly women living in the hotel who "trick" now and then to pay their rent.[5]

The arrangement usually takes place in the bar, with the pimp working out the price. Sexual contacts are in the tenant's room, the whore's "work-bench" (room), or in one of the vacant cars in the hotel parking lot. Most often, they will go to the tenant's room while the girl's pimp waits in the bar. The leniency of the hotel management is an encouragement to the trade, as the "prossies" have little to fear in the way of reprisals, and there is even some deference shown to the "prossies" and their pimps. There is no contempt for a pimp, for, after all, he has a good hustle. The "chippie," on the other hand, who spends all her "trick" money on dope and new clothes for her pimp, is believed to be a real fool, who has a good hustle that she is throwing away so that someone else can make it. The dislike expressed for the "chippie" is related to the greater likelihood of these men having been victimized by them and their pimps. It is not uncommon for a young, inexperienced prostitute to get the man drunk and then call in her pimp, who beats up and robs the old man. When several such beatings occur and the manager begins to anticipate delay in getting his rent money from the victims, the manager initiates a "cleanup" and bans the "prossies" from the hotel. However, since management's overall policy is to ignore the practice, the cleanup is ineffective, and within a few days the situation reverts to normal.

---

could not hold for suspicion of a misdemeanor. Therefore, their "hands are tied."

5. Actually, any woman living in the Guinevere is assumed to be a hooker by the tenants. The evening after I moved into my room, my husband visited. The next morning several people informed the manager that "she had a man in her room." Another incident which occurred several weeks into the field work revealed that for some of the tenants my role in the hotel remained ambiguous. I was sitting with several men in the bar, and one of them (a street peddler in his seventies) offered me ten dollars to sleep with him. Another man became upset, berated him for being insulting to a "high-class broad," and attempted to convince the offender that I was a student writing a book. The street peddler heard him out and then offered me twenty dollars.

Many of the sexual contacts involve "first-of-the-monthers," that is, they occur when the checks arrive. The going rate is ten dollars, rarely more, although some have been known to pay considerably more. "Baldy," a sixty-seven-year-old former fighter, for example, paid sixty dollars for a "blow job." He was, of course, drunk. In terms of actual sexual activity, the following accounts by men in the Guinevere and two prostitutes who work in the area are illuminating:

> All hotels have "prossies"; some hotels have hotel "prossies," and the manager gets a share. They rent a "work-bench" and work right there. They like the old men, well, it's easy money and easy work for them. You have to realize, it's mostly talk. Oh, they'll brag to one another. You can go into the bar and you'll hear them, but that's mostly talk. All this sex talk you hear is just mostly talk.

> It's disgusting. A bunch of "d.g.'s" [sex deviates] here. I keep sex in the corner. I don't mess around with the "prossies." I masturbate, it's just a matter of release.

> The professionals know their business, but them young "chippies" with their pimps and hooked on dope, and they haven't got the brains of a louse.

> It's true, all talk winds up about sex. But, they're really just voyeurs, and the talk is part of that. They pay to look, if you understand me. They pay to look at a young girl, and it's no work for her.

> They don't want much and the money's the same. They like to look and maybe touch, but they don't do much more [a twenty-two-year-old black prostitute].

> It gives 'em something to feel good about. I had a woman, that kinda stuff, and they can tell the others in the bar. Shit, they're just talking, anyway, they're not doin' [a thirty-four-year-old white prostitute].

At any rate, despite the gap between action and talk, the elderly men at the Guinevere appear relatively willing to allow the "prossies" to skim off the tops of their checks. However, it is usually a one-shot affair, as these men have neither the finances nor the desire to maintain women on any permanent basis.

Romances between the elderly tenants are rare—sixty-year-old men do not want sixty-year-old women. When romances do develop, they are short-lived and not a subject of bragging. The men will not bring a lady friend into the bar to show her off and are reticent about such relationships. In the words of one seventy-three-year-old woman, "romances here are torrid and end abruptly, usually over trivia." Long-term relationships between these men and women are precluded by the conflicting demands and expectations referred to earlier. The women attempt to use the relationship as a vehicle to establish a quasi-family situation—the man will be asked to do things for her, to accompany her downtown, to have dinner with her. The man views such expectations as exploitative and possessive on her part. At this point, the relationship usually ends. Several of the men reported prior relationships that they had formed with elderly female tenants, only to have to break them off because the women became too "possessive," "jealous," and "demanding." Since the men define the women as seeking a relationship that they cannot afford and do not want, they prefer the pay-as-you-go services of the prostitute.

For their part, the elderly women define the men as interested only in sex. (They are correct; the liaison with the prostitute constitutes a casual, sharply delimited transaction in which no ongoing demands are made of the relationship.) Involvement with a man is a source of unrelenting gossip, and any friendship between the sexes is always assumed to be a front for the fact that they are sleeping with each other. The strict proscription against "getting too friendly" applies to male-female interaction particularly. Both men and women are inclined to interpret overtures on the part of the other as attempts at exploitation.

The institutionalization of mutual suspicion and avoidance

that characterizes contacts between the elderly men and women has more severe consequences for the women, who must rely on a decreased sociability pool. They do not work and, therefore, do not form work relationships; they do not usually frequent the hotel bar and do not have drinking cronies. And the women, cut off from the company of men, do not relate well to each other either. The attitudes of the women toward each other revolve around the axes of hostility and jealousy. They are in a permanent kind of competition with one another. [6]

Interaction between the women takes the form of one-up-manship, with the goal being to establish that one's family and background are definitely superior to the other. This behavior ought not to be viewed as a feminine counterpart to the "conning" behavior of the hustlers, who are attempting to demonstrate superior abilities over rivals in their occupation. The competition of the hustlers serves as a socially binding force, in that it defines their common interests, skills, and experience. For the women, however, this competitive arena intensifies their bitterness over a life that they cannot leave and cannot live, and drives deep barriers between them.

One informant spoke knowingly of the fragility of relationships between the women:

> Friendships between them [women] never last more than a few days. Then they fall out over some paltry matter. Usually, over gossip. Some of the feuds and vendettas are years old. Friendships between the men are more permanent because they are hard-headed and practical. They need each other for their work. Luther [a

6. We see here, in sharp relief, one of the products of culturally engendered sex-role identities. Women in our society define themselves in terms of their men: when they have no man, they must look upon all other women as rivals for the man they must somehow get to validate their status. These elderly women, who in all probability are not going to get men, nevertheless continue to play out the cultural mandate. They continue to define other women as their competitors and are, as are most women in our society, crippled in their capacity to relate to each other independently of the male-female configuration.

carny boss], now how could he take care of all that by himself? No, he's got to have someone he will know for sure is going to be there; he's got to have his workers. He makes a lot of contacts and holds on to them. But, the women, they're so out of touch with the mainstream. The men don't have anything to do with them. Well, because they can see that they're just interested in using them. Do this for me; oh, won't you drive me there? And, of course, the women are quite boring; they live in the past. Not like the men, who have to keep up with the times. But to get back to the women, no, I don't know any of them who have stayed friends. Friends? They're too jealous and suspicious of one another, always gossiping and backbiting on each other. And sooner or later, it gets back, and there you are, they're not speaking anymore.

All in all, one cannot help being struck by the poignant appearance of these taciturn and suspicious ladies, with their wigs that don't fit and their veiled hats that, like banners, put forth a brave front. Their loneliness and isolation are tangible. Their adoption of an exaggerated unapproachability underscores what is a poorer mastery of the coping strategies needed to make it in the world of the SRO.

The elderly women living in the Guinevere have had to sacrifice more in the way of role identity in order to survive in the SRO world. The giving up of culturally acquired sex-role identities has not been a facile accomplishment, and, indeed, their exaggerated enactment of some of the dominant themes of SRO life—suspicion, avoidance, privacy—are attempts to deal with residual meanings and values, such as dependency and intimacy, that were appropriate to a sex-role identity that no longer is viable. Above all, they are faced with the continual necessity to develop effective coping behaviors.

That there is even less solidarity among these aged women in a group of people distinctive for its impoverishment of social ties is understandable when viewed in the context of the utilitarian and instrumental thrust of relationships established by the SRO tenants. The values of a lifetime, which served to support personal and social identity, are not appropriate in the world of the Guinevere and must be sloughed off. The fracturing of identity that results is the heavy price that these elderly women must pay in order to continue as SRO tenants. They have little choice: they, no less than the men, are locked into their situation by age, poverty, ill health, and their own desire to maintain independence.

CHAPTER EIGHT

"Old Wine"

When I embarked upon this study of elderly SRO tenants, many questions were begging to be answered: What are the social roles available within this society? Which roles are positively valued? What conditions call forth and promote group solidarity? What are the bases for entering into relationships? What are the supportive norms and values that buttress role behaviors? What are the characteristic forms of interaction between the SRO tenants and outsiders? How is deviance managed? What is the range of coping skills? How is selfhood maintained?

In a general way, my findings support previous research in the area. The Guinevere, like other SRO hotels in the deteriorating inner cores of our cities, houses a large proportion of individuals who have personal histories that reflect alienation, deviance, and low degrees of involvement in the conventional institutions of American society. Here live the petty thieves, the alcoholics, the addicts, the hustlers, the unattached urban poor, the down-and-outers. Many of these individuals have been only marginally attached to the normative institutions of family and work throughout the greater part of their adult lives. When they reach the Guinevere, most of them have spent a lifetime working down to the SRO environment. They experienced no sudden, catastrophic event that catapulted them into the atomistic, alienated world of the SRO. Rather, they have gradually but inexorably been settling in for a long time. These are people with tarnished identities. When viewed from the perspective of the larger society, the aged tenants, in their failure to live out cultural mandates, typify the "misfits," the rejects, the "losers."

The SRO population has certain identifiable characteristics —higher proportion of single individuals, extreme poverty, concentration of physical and mental handicaps. Many of these individuals have life spaces that are grossly restricted, often extending no farther than the narrow confines of their rooms, the hotel bar, the hotel lobby. Their efforts and energies are narrowed so as to encompass only immediate, personal needs. For them, the horizon is the next social security check. The locked-in nature of their life style is assured by the twin determinants of low rent and low income. Dominant features of the world of the SRO, as we have seen, include severe forms of isolation and depersonalization, and the institutionalization of mutual suspicion.

The elderly tenants at the Guinevere are not linked up into a cohesive social community; relationships are always problematic. These people are truly "loners." They have broken all ties to family and friends, and, for the most part, do not attempt to replenish what was already an impoverished repertoire of social relationships.[1] They live in a world marked by the extremes of alienation, isolation, and anonymity.

The task of adequately interpreting the profile of the SRO society that emerges from this study involves two interrelated issues: on the one hand, these people maintain social relationships that are fragile, problematic, and susceptible to change and dissolution; and, on the other hand, they are very adept at manipulating relationships when social ties will serve their

1. The majority of these individuals have always been to some degree "loners" and do not find SRO society strange or discordant with their previous life styles. For a preliminary discussion of extreme lifelong isolates and morale, see two articles by Lowenthal: "Social Isolation and Mental Illness in Old Age" and "Interaction and Adaptation."

purposes. The ability to understand these findings is dependent upon the methodological stance, which has allowed a view from within. As a participating observer, I learned and took part in the taken-for-granted meanings that the residents of the Guinevere construct and which, in turn, underpin behaviors.[2] As I entered into their world of meanings, I began to depart significantly from certain major trends in social gerontology. That these elderly men and women eschew the company of each other and live markedly isolated lives cannot be explained away by recourse to variants of the "aging process" theme, which puts forth the position that some mysterious process called "aging" stands over and above situated features and will, somehow, make interpretive sense of data on old people. Such a position is repudiated by the findings of this study.

The gerontological literature emphasizes the return to dependency and passivity allegedly characteristic of the elderly. No doubt the picture of what it means to be old in America in the twentieth century that emerges from these studies is distorted by the overreliance upon institutionalized aged as the subjects for much of the research. Institutionalized elderly *are* passive, terrified, and dependent, and they do slip away irrevocably from the world of the living:

> Old Wine: Grandpa's Dead
> Night rider, moon rider
> Black rose of latticed porches
> and musty attics
> Took the old man
> sit sitting
> among his over-stuffed upholstery flowers
> with a white-haired whimper.
> No one listened, no one heard
> the tin-pan clatter
> of rushing winter leaves.
>   [Robert Lewis Stephens]

2. See the methodological appendix, pp. 101-9.

However, the Guinevere tenants do not belong with the old man, excluded from society, sitting and waiting to die in his overstuffed upholstery flowers, for they are actively involved in the perpetuation of their society. The fragmented nature of the Guinevere society is continually reasserted and reconstructed in an active manner by these people. They are not passive victims of old age; they are alienated and alone, but not because "disengagement" is one of those behaviors that accompanies aging. Rather, their reality, which they have constructed and within which they live, can be penetrated and survived only by individuals acting alone in their own self-interest. Interpersonal bonds are vehicles to be utilized when they facilitate the achievement of these individual goals, and handicaps to be avoided when they do not serve. The isolation, anonymity, and suspicion endemic to the world of our SRO tenants are not accidental byproducts of urban conditions or old age; they are, however, the deliberate consequences of the active participation of these slum dwellers in the structuring of their social reality and, as such, are instruments to deal with the exigencies of this reality.

They have a well-developed capacity to handle interpersonal losses and gains; they are isolates because it serves their interests, and they come together to establish social bonds when individual goals will be better served by the instrumentality of relationships. The form of the relationships is utilitarian, nonintimate, economic, in short, a kind of negotiated exchange. Relationships are based on a *quid pro quo* standard: they are cold-blooded, calculated affairs designed to accomplish specific individual ends.

Lines of demarcation defining the obligations of roles are clearly drawn so that violations of dominant themes of privacy, independence, suspicion are kept to a minimum. As an example, one recalls the isolating of the women when they violate these expectations.

In the SRO world, individuals act as individuals, pursuing personal goals with only the minimum of consensual norms. In the SRO, individuals survive at the expense of larger social groupings. As noted previously, the exception of the carnies, who have managed to develop a continuing network of relationships, rests on the special requirements of the hustling trade.

These old ghetto dwellers are literally surrounded by hostile forces, from muggers to exploitative shopkeepers to other tenants who, like themselves, are busy looking out for Number One. Their construction of reality, with its shared assumptions as to the meanings of events, represents their attempt to cope with this harsh environment. The coping strategies that are elaborated into normative mandates are efficient in promoting their efforts to get by, to make it.

That the majority are forced to utilize all available energy and resources to wrest from a noxious environment even the basic necessities is, of course, unalterably connected to their need for and inability to realize physical security. The norms demanding avoidance of close ties (which would render the individual vulnerable) enable these elderly people to anticipate and then mobilize to meet potentially destructive events and situations. A primary coping skill is an active policy of noninvolvement.

The strategies devised by these elderly tenants to deal with deviance evoke another facet to the "losers" versus "survivors" dialectic. They react to deviance emanating from outside their midst by implementing behaviors reflective of the dominant norms, but to deviance emanating from within their midst, they display a remarkable tolerance. This tolerance is a dramatic example of their own efforts to cope with another basic dilemma—that of managing and sustaining an acceptable social identity. Contrary to stereotypes about the aged, we have found these elderly people to be flexible in their capacity to tolerate change, disorder, unconventionality, and loss. These people are not passive and they are not "nice": they are tough, and they are persistent. But most of all, they are survivors.

The importance of the hustle underscores the extremely

marginal status of these people. As one of the carnies remarked, "Everyone here has a hustle." The intense preoccupation with the hustle is only a specific instance of the larger issue which concerns all of our Guinevere tenants, namely, getting by, coping, making it.

The changing impressions which I experienced during my field work were both instructive and prophetic. Initially, the world of the Guinevere seemed exceedingly strange—it was highly depersonalized, and there was an atmosphere of anonymity pervaded by a sense of transiency, despite the fact that many of the residents have been there for years. The Guinevere tenants seemed such a sorry lot of losers and down-and-outers, who were hostile and demoralized. And so it was, until they allowed me entrance into their world of meanings and experiences.

In the final stages of field work, the intimate knowledge that I was able to glean from living with these people and coming to understand their constructed meanings necessitated the rejection of those initial impressions and judgments. The independence, the insistence upon privacy and dignity, the sheer tenacity of these people must invoke a considerable respect. The "oldtimers" at the Guinevere are making it in an environment in which everyone is a potential exploiter, a potential threat. There is no one they can trust—no family, no friends. There is only oneself. That they react by passivity does not mean that they are passive; that they choose not to respond to overtures is not to be interpreted as another case of regression in the aged. What is myopically defined as regression, passivity, acquiescence, incompetence in the tendency of old people to nonresponse must be interpreted from a different perspective—from the "other side." If we do this, we will be able to "know of" the world of the aged SRO tenant, and we will come to understand how their behavior is an aggressive, active stance against a hostile environment. But we cannot understand this until and unless we are able to enter into their world of meanings.

So, let us have done with the tendency in gerontology to assign to some vaguely defined process called "aging" the reasons for what elderly people do and do not. Rather, let us look at specific populations of elderly men and women in their natural settings—whether it be the SRO hotel, a suburban apartment, a retirement village in Phoenix City—and get to the business of studying the situated aspects of human behavior.

To this end, the aging hustlers at the Guinevere can tell us of the vicissitudes of their mode of adjustment to the world of the SRO. This adjustment is made in the face of powerful odds against them, not the least of which are those very agencies and practitioners whose ostensible task it is to service these people. The professional "doers of good deeds" cannot expect realistically to gain the cooperation of these people. Why ought they to risk the subversion of those values and norms that permit the survival of a life style which, at least, allows them their own kind of old age? How dare they be required to become vulnerable? The service agencies are not their friends; at best, they are ineffective and neutral, and at worst, their tamperings seriously interfere with the fragile balance whose preservation demands such hard work. The armament of survival strategies of these people has withstood the harshest tests: they are the real survivors. A seventy-six-year-old man who has been living at the hotel for eleven years put it all together: "If they'd just leave me alone. I'm happy here. I do what I want. I'm okay, I've had a good life, and I don't owe anybody a damned thing."

Postscript

Loners, Losers, and Lovers began as my research effort to satisfy the requirements for the Ph.D. As a teaching assistant in the Sociology Department of a large midwestern university, I had grown tired of participating in the familiar university custom of teaching all those interminable "discussion groups" for introductory sociology, while others in the upper echelons divided up the department spoils and were free to teach graduate seminars and do research. I had also grown tired of starving on the pittance reluctantly doled out to those in this lowly status. The union card, euphemistically termed a doctor of philosophy degree, was a necessity, and so I embarked on my dissertation research.

But somewhere in the course of realizing this study, the scenario changed, and with it the meaning of this endeavor. The instrument of this change was the research experience itself, and gradually my singleminded goal of completing academic requirements began to seem slightly tarnished and more than a little selfish. I think that I shall never be the same person who entered the world of the SRO tenant. The experience shook up my commitments and my priorities, and dealt a lethal blow to the myth of scientific "objectivity" which I, along with my peers, had accepted without much question.

The world of the SRO is closed to outsiders—hostile to social workers, resistant to scientific intruders, and contemptuous of compassionate do-gooders. That the SRO residents tolerated and eventually came to accept me is remarkable enough, and a gift for which I am thankful. They did not have to let me in. Their own normative system forbade such brash intrusions into their secrets, and I could offer them little in the way of recompense. Nevertheless, they did grant entrance and even acceptance, and to them I owe the intellectual and emotional adventure that *Loners, Losers, and Lovers* was to become.

Perhaps fieldworkers are often changed by their research experience, perhaps even usually this is the case. I don't know. The literature on field work experiences is frustratingly coy about this issue. Be that as it may, such was my case, and if I seem unduly euphoric about it, then I will just have to be forgiven.

Researchers do not walk into the field *tabula rasa,* they carry with them the appurtenances of prior socialization, including the internalized norms peculiar to academia. Most likely, they have steeped themselves in the literature on their chosen subject. My preparation for research followed this time-honored pattern. But I was to have prior stereotypes (for such they turned out to be) shaken and even devastated by the reality that confronted me. To mention one cultural myth that was shattered, the "old-timers" in the SRO world violated canons of passivity and dependence. Passivity and dependency are ascriptive roles reserved for the old in our society, and the social science literature has produced little that might lead us to question these cultural mandates. The elderly SRO tenants betray us. They are not passive and dependent; they are mean and tough, and neither give quarter nor ask for quarter. Where passivity seemed to be a characteristic response on their part, further probing revealed that it was merely a mask for an aggressive stance which used the appearance of passivity in a deliberate and manipulative fashion. Dependency was despised as a cardinal sin in the SRO world. As for the mellow grandmotherly and grandfatherly "types," they are not to be found in the

SRO society.

After two months in the SRO world, I said, in my naïveté, "These people are real losers; theirs is a world of isolation and the end of hopes and desires." But later, the inaccuracy of this judgment was to become all too clear. These scarred residents in our cities' rotting cores are, in fact, the real survivors. That they are surviving on their own terms is a tribute to their ingenuity, their tenacity, and their courage.

Methodological Appendix

The methodology of this research was influenced greatly by three goals formulated in the planning stage of the study: to conduct naturalistic research by observing a "selected portion of everyday life"; to develop a thorough descriptive analysis of the social world of the aged residents of an SRO hotel; and to contribute to sociological theory through the generation of grounded theory in the substantive area of aging.

The decision to obtain observations *in situ* instead of using alternate data-collection procedures grew out of a preference for symbolic interactionism as an orienting theoretical framework.[1] Symbolic interactionism embraces a methodology of direct observation of the empirical world; thus, I chose to utilize a methodology that would permit observation in the most immediate way of relevant data on the aged SRO tenant.

Symbolic interactionism theory rejects behavioristic explanations of social behavior, which tend to be mechanistic in character and to assume externality in assigning cause to the study of behavioral events. Symbolic interactionism assumes that behavior is self-directed and observable at two distinct levels—

1. I refer to symbolic interactionism as formulated and developed by such seminal thinkers as John Dewey, George Herbert Mead, Charles Horton Cooley, and, more recently, Herbert Blumer, Howard S. Becker, Erving Goffman, and Harold Garfinkel.

the symbolic and the interactional. Analysis must capture the symbolic meanings that emerge over time in interaction. These symbols are "manifold, complex, verbal, nonverbal, intended, unintended."[2] Herbert Blumer, criticizing approaches that treat social interaction as merely the medium through which determining factors produce behavior, indicates that all social objects of study are "interpreted" by individuals and thus have social meaning. This process of interpretation ("defining the situation") is inherent in the human condition and our understanding of it.

Symbolic interactionism contains a methodological preference, namely, a method that lays stress upon "feeling one's way inside the experience of the actor."[3] Herbert Blumer has advised conducting "naturalistic" research, which is better equipped to cope with the situated aspects of human social behavior. For social research, the empirical world must be the central point of concern. The "obdurate" character of the empirical world more readily yields up its secrets to the direct examination of social behavior and interaction in everyday, natural settings. Thus, the research protocol most compatible with symbolic interaction theory involves selecting areas for study on the level of common experience, that is, observations from a selected portion of everyday life. Further, studies guided by symbolic interaction theory tend to use observation rather than experimentation under artificially controlled conditions. Thus, a thorough descriptive analysis, as opposed to a reductive analysis (which tends to result from data gathered in a radically simplified setting), was a goal which to a large degree specified the advantages of particular methodological procedures.

Participant observation was the primary means of data collection. The researcher assumed the role of participant-as-observer. The role of complete participant was neither feasible nor, in my judgment, ethically defensible. During various activ-

2. Denzin, *The Research Act*, p. 7.
3. Manis and Meltzer, eds., *Symbolic Interaction*, p. 1.

ities, I switched to the role of complete observer, for example, during heavy drinking bouts of social groupings in the hotel bar, while observing the interaction of manager and tenants, during situations of violence, or in situations where changes in activity were initiated by group members. When I was not competent to participate effectively and would not have been expected to by the subjects, and when I did not wish to influence group changes and decisions, I temporarily assumed the complete observer role.[4]

The participant-as-observer role was defined early in the course of the study; it permitted more ready acceptance by the tenants and staff of the Guinevere. In addition, the clear assumption of this role promoted the reciprocal processes of informant training and the subjects' educating of me to the norms and values of their world. Reactions to me as researcher evolved through a discernible pattern—from initial skepticism to an earnest desire that I "get everything and not miss anything." During the first days of field work I was hesitant to record observations publicly and relied upon memory to record observations and events after they occurred. However, as the reason for my being in the hotel became known and accepted, on-the-spot recording was soon possible and even comfortable. During the course of conversations and interviews, the subjects often asked me such questions as, "Did you get that, are you sure that you got all that?" On one occasion, while gathering detailed information on the techniques of hawking balloons and plastic novelties from some of the tenants who make their living street vending, I was gently chastised by the subjects for not writing down everything they said. Thus, the collection of data was facilitated by the reciprocal process of role defining initiated by the fieldworker and participated in by the subjects.

In addition to participant observation, I utilized several other techniques for gathering data, including informant interviewing, taped interviews, analysis of hotel documents, and

4. For a full discussion of the roles available to the fieldworker, see Gold, "Roles in Sociological Field Observations."

unobtrusive measures. Because participant observation is not a single technique but rather involves the use of a variety of techniques of data collection which increases the sources and types of data, it was possible to exercise great flexibility and scope in pursuing possible categories of data. I effected a triangulation of methods—specifically, triangulation of data, triangulation of subjects, and triangulation of techniques. The use of multi-measurement was deemed essential to provide for: (1) the widest scope in obtaining relevant data; (2) an ongoing and rigorous means of cross-validation and counterchecks of emergent findings; and (3) the checking out of the adequacy and accuracy of data by utilizing measurement techniques whose differing strengths and weaknesses would function as mutual checks on each other.[5]

The triangulation of data-collection techniques provided a means of establishing confidence in the findings and of refining hypotheses as they were formulated during the course of field work. An example of this advantage was the analysis of hotel records, which permitted ready access to a wealth of material that would have taken months to gather through interviews and, in addition, was less subject to error. The use of the taped interview served to focus on specific issues that needed clarification. The use of unobtrusive measures introduced "nonreactive" means of observation, and were additional sources of data that held little possibility of bias. Two illustrations of unobtrusive measures used are: counting of bar receipts to confirm the observation that the amount of patronage increased at the first and middle of the month, and analysis of the hotel records which, known only to the manager, permitted access to sensitive data. These findings were then cross-checked against data gathered by the other, more traditional means.[6]

5. The rationale behind multi-measurement (triangulation) has been presented by a number of authors. See Denzin, *Research Act*; Webb, "Unconventionality, Triangulation, and Inference"; and Phillips, *Knowledge from What?*

6. For a discussion of the types and advantages of "nonreactive" measures

Triangulation of subjects was effected as observations, conversations, interviews, and activities were recorded with tenants, management, staff, social workers, service personnel to the hotel (mailmen, police, fumigators), the owners of cafes, novelty shops, markets, and so forth, in the areas that are frequented by the subjects, and some tenants and staff personnel of nearby SRO hotels. This procedure of seeking comparison groups was crucial in determining whether the findings of the target group in the Guinevere could be generalized to a larger population.

I maintained a daily log in which I recorded observations, conversations, interviews, events, impressions, and tentative interpretations. I was very careful to differentiate observed data from impressions and interpretations. All entries were identified at the time of entry with regard to time, date, setting, and persons involved. This was essential as the volume of field entries grew. At the end of each day's observations, I examined the entries for the day and added any material that might have been omitted; I was careful to see that this recall data was differentiated from on-the-spot recorded data. The listing of source, time, place—in other words, the context of entries—proved invaluable as the process of collecting, organizing, and analyzing data continued.

The voluminous body of field notes required an indexing system, which was periodically revised as significant areas of interest began to form. This indexing of data was gradually expanded into a cross indexing of entries about midway through the course of the field work, as the interrelationships of observations demanded a more complex system.

The analysis of the findings was sequential and ongoing during the entire course of the research. Thus, the generation of relevant categories and their properties, the formulation of hypotheses, the search for comparison groups were not activities which had definite beginnings and endings denoting dis-

in social research, see Webb *et al.*, *Unobtrusive Measures*; Phillips, *Knowledge from What?*; and Denzin, *Research Act*.

tinct stages of the research. It is axiomatic that the method utilized demanded the continual reformulation and refinement of research hypotheses, that they might correspond more closely to the empirical data and express more accurately the general relationships among the derived data.

I was guided by the contention that field-work data are not merely "impressionistic," but are conducive to the discovery of concepts and hypotheses that, having been derived from the data, are singularly resistant to invalidation. Glaser and Strauss, in their discussion of the strategy of discovering and generating *grounded* theory, point out that much of current sociological research is geared toward the verification of existing theory through data, and that the generation of theory from data (grounded theory) has been neglected.[7] They argue that theory grounded in data is less vulnerable to refutation than theory deduced from a priori assumptions. Grounded theory fits the data and works, having been generated from the data itself, whereas theory based on logical speculation and not generated from empirical data often does not fit—with the result of "forcing" the data—and does not explain as adequately. A further ramification of their argument, of course, is that we ought to abandon the current tendency to separate theory from methods, and acknowledge their essential relationship.

The strategy of generating theory from data involves the realization that qualitative data are not merely explorative or impressionistic, but are also generative, in that the concepts and their properties which constitute the elementary units in theoretical paradigms are derived directly from the data (rather than imposed from without by a priori deductive schemas), and correspond closely to the "real" (empirical) world. It follows that the generalized relations (hypotheses) developed from these empirically derived conceptual categories are more likely

7. For an understanding of the logic and method of grounded theory, see the writings of Glaser and Strauss listed in the bibliography. See also Denzin, *Research Act,* and the same author's introduction to part 3 of his *Sociological Methods.*

to stand up to the rigorous testing and verification essential to the validation of research findings. Thus, grounded theory is especially fruitful in making theoretical contributions because the process by which it was generated demands that it closely fit the substantive area in which it is to be used.

Viewing the development of grounded theory as a *process* of building theory from data provides the researcher with appropriate and powerful protocols for accomplishing the necessary steps in any research enterprise, that is, collecting the data, organizing it, analyzing it, and interpreting the meanings of observations. The method of generating grounded theory utilized in this study of SRO aged demanded an ongoing system of built-in controls and checks on these steps to assure confidence in the findings.

The goal of generating grounded theory further necessitated a constant comparative method. As relevant categories were derived from the data, certain core categories were defined; a progressive building up of conceptual categories and their properties led to hypotheses which stated the interrelationships of these categories. The categories and hypotheses were tested by seeking out comparison groups, and determining the degree of accuracy and generality of the proposed explanations. To obtain maximum depth and density, it was essential that the core categories be saturated.[8]

The major advantages of utilizing this method of theory development lay in the practical consequences of viewing theory construction as a process which must focus the attention of the researcher on a particular substantive area and simultaneously

8. In contrast to the method of analytic induction, the constant comparison method does not require complete coverage of the whole area under study (except at the beginning when main categories are emerging). Rather, it requires the saturation of data on categories that are necessary for the generation of hypotheses. For treatments of the method of analytic induction, see Znaniecki, *The Method of Sociology*; Becker *et al.*, *Boys in White*; Cressey, *Other People's Money*; Lindesmith, *Addiction and Opiates*; Robinson, "The Logical Structure of Analytic Induction"; and Turner, "The Quest for Universals in Sociological Research."

determine the scope and direction of the research act. Thus, during all phases of this research study, both theory and method worked together to determine the types of data sought, the classification of data into conceptual categories, the formulation of hypotheses, and the integration of these into a framework. The ongoing and dynamic character of this method provided internal checks on the key problems in evaluating findings, namely, problems of proof, inference, validity, reliability, and generalizability.

The contributions of any research study must be weighed in conjunction with the limitations of the particular research. The shortcomings of this research are undeniable—a real shortage of funds set boundaries on both equipment and time; a team approach, as a further guarantee of the triangulation of data-collection procedures, would have been preferable; it is likely that more comparative data on other SRO hotels could have resulted in the refinement and modification of my conclusions. The shortcomings and unanswered questions of this study point the way toward future research on the urban aged. I suggest, specifically, a study of the relationship between chronic alcoholism and the practice of "jungling up" that is found in certain SRO populations. Of great interest would be an investigation into the movement patterns of these elderly poor as they shift from one hotel to another. We are in need of case studies of the elderly women in SROs, that we may delineate the distinguishing features of their personal careers which deviate so markedly from those of the majority of aged women in our society. There is a need for research into hustling as a primary work situation for marginal groups in our society. We would profit by the development of hustling taxonomies from which comparisons could be taken and the degree of overlap established. Certainly, we are urgently in need of research which is longitudinal in design and can spell out the life careers of the SRO elderly. The sociologist must experience frustration when confronted with the gaps in systematic knowledge on marginal groups, of which the aged slum dweller is one. Research is urgently needed into the condition of the urban, aged poor; and the above are only a few representative issues to which we must begin to address ourselves.

List of Terms Used by the Carnies

Agent: a pimp.

B.C.: be careful.

Bird-dog: tenants' term for other tenants and hotel staff who spy on them and report to the hotel manager.

C note: one hundred dollars.

Carnese: carny talk, a mixture of pig latin and underworld slang.

Carnies: peddlers, so called because of their use of carnese and prior association with carnivals and circuses.

Carriage trade: sales made to passing cars.

Case: to scrutinize, from the viewpoint of judging how much money one can make.

Century: one hundred dollars.

Chippie: young prostitute on narcotics, an inexperienced prostitute.

Chill: to become suspicious.

Come out: a large turnout of people for an event, their willingness to spend freely.

Con: to tell a good story, to put someone on; also, a type of hustle.

Cover the stock: to sell enough to equal the investment in merchandise.

Dime: ten dollars.

Dummy up: to be quiet.

Elbow-bending: drinking.

Fin: five dollars.

First-of-the-monthers: elderly men who have prostitutes on the first of the month, when their social security checks arrive.

Flash: showy, up-front merchandise.

Gandy-dancer: operator of a concession selling novelties.

Geedus: money.

Gestapo: police.

Go-for: person who earns money by getting cigarettes, alcohol, and the like for someone; a type of hustle.

Grab joint: a hamburger stand.

Grouch bag: pouches worn by vendors in which they keep their change.

Half a yard: fifty dollars.

LIST OF TERMS USED BY THE CARNIES

Hard: coins.

Hawker: street vendor.

Heat: the law, pressure from any source.

High line: expensive stock.

Ho: to hold out for a larger amount of money.

Homeguard: local, competing concessions.

Hustle: general term including a variety of unconventional, marginal ways of earning a living, for example, peddling, begging, go-fors, etc.; ways of earning a living for someone who cannot find steady employment.

Hustler: one who has a hustle, sometimes used synonymously with peddler.

Jump a girl: sexual intercourse.

Jungling up: several tenants cook and eat communal meals.

Kelsy: a woman on a cash basis.

Larry: damaged, useless stock.

Lines: money.

Low line: cheap, unappealing stock.

Lunch bag: homosexual term, refers to an athletic supporter.

Mark: a customer; broadly, anyone who is not a hustler.

Moola: money.

Outsider: refers to people who do not live in SRO hotels; sometimes used to refer to transients in SROs broadly, anyone who is not a permanent resident; a nonhustler, a customer.

P.C.: percentage.

Pipe that beetle: look at the girl.

Privilege: place where a peddler sets up his stall and displays his wares.

Professional: prostitute who is experienced.

Prossie: prostitute.

Rag pickers: police.

Riding academy: hotel or motel catering predominantly to prostitutes.

Round easy: turn around slowly and look at someone.

Roscoe: hand gun.

Rubbers: balloons.

Runners: go-fors.

Scratch: money.

Scuff: barely to make a living.

Soft: bills.

Sponsor: a pimp.

Squeeze: canned heat (Sterno) squeezed through a sock or a pillowcase then diluted with water and drunk by skid-row alcoholics.

Stable: several prostitutes working for a pimp.

Take it on the Arthur Dufy: go away.

There's a herring in the place: there's an outsider asking questions.

Work bench: rooms rented by prostitutes.

Yard: one hundred dollars.

Bibliography

Aaronson, Bernard S. "Personality Stereotypes of Aging." *Journal of Gerontology* 21 (1966):458-62.

Adams, Richard N., and Preiss, Jack J., eds. *Human Organization Research, Field Relations and Techniques*. Homewood, Ill.: The Dorsey Press, 1960.

Anderson, Nels. *The Hobo*. Chicago: University of Chicago Press, 1923.

Argyis, Chris. "Diagnosing Defenses Against the Outsider." *Journal of Social Issues* 8 (1952):24-34.

Barron, Milton L. "Minority Group Characteristics of the Aged in American Society." *Journal of Gerontology* 8 (1953): 477-81.

Becker, Howard S. *Outsiders: Studies in the Sociology of Deviance*. New York: The Free Press, 1963.

Becker, Howard S., and Geer, Blanche. "Participant Observation and Interviewing: A Comparison." *Human Organization* 16 (1957):28-32.

Becker, Howard S., Geer, Blanche, Hughes, Everett C., and Strauss, Anselm L. *Boys in White: Student Culture in Medical School*. Chicago: University of Chicago Press, 1961.

Bekker, L. DeMoyne, and Taylor, Charles. "Attitudes Toward the Aged in a Multi-generational Sample." *Journal of Gerontology* 21 (1966):115-18.

Bell, Tony. "The Relationship Between Social Involvement and Feeling Old Among Residents in Homes for the Aged." *Journal of Gerontology* 22 (1967):17-22.

Benney, Mark, and Hughes, Everett C. "Of Sociology and the Interview: Editorial Preface." *American Journal of Sociology* 62 (1956):137-42.

Blau, Zena Smith. "Changes in Status and Age Identification." *American Sociological Review* 21 (1956):198-203.

Bloom, K. L. "Age and the Self-Concept." *American Journal of Psychiatry* 118 (1961):534-38.

Blumer, Herbert. *Symbolic Interactionism: Perspective and Method*. Englewood Cliffs, N.J.: Prentice-Hall, 1969.

113

————. "What is Wrong with Social Theory?" *American Sociological Review* 19 (1954):3-10.

Bogue, Donald J. *Skidrow in American Cities.* Chicago: University of Chicago Press, 1963.

Britton, Joseph H. "Dimensions of Adjustment of Older Adults." *Journal of Gerontology* 18 (1963):60-65.

Bucher, Rue, Fritz, Charles E., and Quarantelli, E. L. "Tape Recorded Interviews in Social Research." *American Sociological Review* 21 (1956):359-64.

Bultena, Gordon L. "Life Continuity and Morale in Old Age." *The Gerontologist* 9 (1969):251-53.

Burgess, Ernest, ed. *Aging in Western Societies: A Comparative Survey.* Chicago: University of Chicago Press, 1940.

————, ed. *The Urban Community.* University of Chicago Sociological Series. Chicago: University of Chicago Press, 1926.

Butler, Robert. "Age-Ism: Another Form of Bigotry." *The Gerontologist* 9 (1969):243-46.

Camilleri, Santo F. "Theory, Probability, and Induction in Social Research." *American Sociological Review* 27 (1962): 170-78.

Caplow, Theodore. "The Dynamics of Information Interviewing." *American Journal of Sociology* 62 (1956):165-71.

Carp, Frances. "Attitudes of Older Persons Toward Themselves and Toward Others." *Journal of Gerontology* 22 (1967):308-12.

————. "Differences Among Older Workers, Volunteers, and Persons Who Are Neither." *Journal of Gerontology* 23 (1968):308-12.

————. "The Mobility of Older Slum-dwellers." *The Gerontologist* 12 (1972):57-65.

Clark, Margaret, and Anderson, Barbara. *Culture and Aging: An Anthropological Study of Older Americans.* Springfield, Ill.: Charles C. Thomas, 1967.

Cressey, Donald R. *Other People's Money.* Glencoe, Ill.: The Free Press, 1953.

Cumming, Elaine, and Henry, William. *Growing Old.* New York: Basic Books, 1961.

Curtin, Sharon R. *Nobody Ever Died of Old Age.* Boston: Little, Brown, 1972.

Denzin, Norman K. *The Research Act.* Chicago: Aldine Publishing Co., 1970.

————, ed. *Sociological Methods.* Chicago: Aldine Publishing Co., 1970.

Dinitz, Simon, Dynes, Russell R., and Clarke, Alfred C., eds. *Deviance: Studies in the Process of Stigmatization and Societal Reaction.* New York: Oxford University Press, 1969.

Glaser, Barney G., and Strauss, Anselm L. *Awareness of Dying.* Chicago: Aldine Publishing Co., 1965.

————. "Discovery of Grounded Theory." *American Behavioral Scientist* 8 (1965):5-11.

————. *The Discovery of Grounded Theory.* Chicago: Aldine Publishing Co., 1967.

————. "Discovery of Substantive Theory: A Basic Strategy for Underlying

Qualitative Research." *Human Organization* 8 (1965): 5-12.

Goffman, Erving. *Stigma: Notes on the Management of Spoiled Identity.* Englewood Cliffs, N.J.: Prentice-Hall, 1963.

Gold, Raymond L. "Roles in Sociological Field Observations." *Social Forces* 36 (1958):217-23.

Habenstein, Robert W., ed. *Pathways to Data.* Chicago: Aldine Publishing Co., 1970.

Hammond, Phillip E., ed. *Sociologists at Work: Essays on the Craft of Social Research.* New York: Basic Books, 1964.

Havighurst, Robert, and Albrecht, Ruth. *Older People.* New York: Longmans Publishing Co., 1953.

Hayner, Norman S. *Hotel Life.* Chapel Hill: University of North Carolina Press, 1936.

Heilbrun, Alfred, and Lair, Charles. "Decreased Role Consistency in the Aged: Implications for Behavioral Pathology." *Journal of Gerontology* 19 (1964):325-29.

Henry, Jules. *Culture Against Man.* New York: Vintage Books, 1963.

Hughes, Everett Cherrington. *Men and Their Work.* Glencoe: The Free Press, 1958.

Jacobs, Glenn, ed. *The Participant Observer.* New York: George Braziller, 1970.

Jacobs, Jerry, ed. *Getting By: Illustrations of Marginal Living.* Boston: Little, Brown, 1973.

Jahoda, Marie, Deutsch, Morton, and Cook, Stuart W., eds. *Research Methods in Social Relations.* New York: The Dryden Press, 1951.

James, William. "A Study of the Expression of Bodily Posture." *Journal of General Psychology* 7 (1932):405-37.

Kastenbaum, Robert, ed. *Contributions to the Psycho-Biology of Aging.* New York: Springer Publishing Co., 1965.

————, ed. *New Thoughts on Old Age.* New York: Springer Publishing Co., 1964.

Kolaja, Jiri. "A Contribution to the Theory of Participant Observation." *Social Forces* 35 (1956):159-63.

Lawton, M. Powell, and Kleban, Morton H. "The Aged Resident of the Inner City." *The Gerontologist* 11 (1971):277-83.

Lawton, M. Powell, Kleban, Morton H., and Singer, Maurice. "The Aged Jewish Person and the Slum Environment." *Journal of Gerontology* 26 (1971):231-39.

Lenzer, Anthony, Pond, Adele S., and Scott, John. *Michigan's Older People: Six Hundred Thousand Over Sixty-Five.* Ann Arbor: State of Michigan, Legislative Advisory Council on Problems of the Aging, 1958.

Lindesmith, Alfred R. *Addiction and Opiates.* Chicago: Aldine Publishing Co., 1968.

Loether, Herman J. *Problems of Aging.* Belmont, Calif.: Dickenson Publishing Co., 1967.

Lowenthal, Marjorie Fiske. "Social Isolation and Mental Illness in Old Age." *American Sociological Review* 29 (1964):54-70.

BIBLIOGRAPHY

Lowenthal, Marjorie Fiske, and Haven, Clayton. "Interaction and Adaptation: Intimacy as a Critical Variable." *American Sociological Review* 33 (1968):20-30.

McCall, George J., and Simmons, J. L., eds. *Issues in Participant Observation: A Text and Reader.* Reading, Mass.: Addison-Wesley, 1969.

Maddox, George, and Eisdorfer, Carl. "Some Correlates of Activity and Morale Among the Elderly." *Social Forces* 40 (1962): 254-60.

Manis, Jerome G., and Meltzer, Bernard N., eds. *Symbolic Interaction: A Reader in Social Psychology.* Boston: Allyn and Bacon, 1967.

Mason, Evelyn. "Some Correlates of Self-judgments of the Aged." *Journal of Gerontology* 9 (1954):324-37.

Mead, George H. *Mind, Self, and Society.* Chicago: University of Chicago Press, 1934.

Meltzer, H. "Age Differences in Happiness and Life Adjustments of Workers." *Journal of Gerontology* 18 (1963):66-70.

Miller, S. J. "The Social Dilemma of the Aging Leisure Participant." In *Older People and Their Social World,* edited by Arnold M. Rose and Warren Peterson, pp. 77-92. Philadelphia: F. A. Davis, 1965.

Myrdal, Gunnar. *Objectivity in Social Research.* New York: Pantheon Books, 1969.

Niebanck, Paul L., with the assistance of John B. Pope. *The Elderly in Older Urban Areas.* Philadelphia: Institute for Environmental Studies, University of Pennsylvania, 1965.

Olesen, Virginia L., and Whittaker, Elvi Waik. "Role-making in Participant Observation: Processes in the Researcher-actor Relationship." *Human Organization* 26 (1967):273-81.

Park, Robert Ezra. *Human Communities.* Glencoe, Ill.: The Free Press, 1952.

Payne, Raymond. "Some Theoretical Approaches to the Sociology of Aging." *Social Forces* 38 (1960):359-62.

Pettit, Lois. "Aged and Alone in Detroit: Summary and Conclusions of a Three-part Study in Health and Welfare Needs of the Aged Living in Detroit's Central Area." Mimeographed. Detroit: Neighborhood Service Organizations, 1962.

Phillips, Derek L. *Knowledge from What?* Chicago: Rand McNally, 1971.

Polsky, Ned. *Hustlers, Beats, and Others.* New York: Doubleday, Anchor Books, 1969.

Preston, Caroline. "A Measure of Self-perception Among Older People." *Journal of Gerontology* 21 (1966):63-67.

———. "Subjectively Perceived Agedness and Retirement." *Journal of Gerontology* 23 (1968):201-4.

———. "Traits Endorsed by Older Non-retired and Retired Subjects." *Journal of Gerontology* 21 (1966):261-64.

Redfield, Robert. "The Art of Social Science." *American Journal of Sociology* 54 (1948):181-90.

Riley, Matilda W. "Social Gerontology and the Age Stratification of Society." Paper read at the Gerontological Society Annual Meeting, 30 October 1970, at Toronto, Ontario. Mimeographed.

Robinson, W. S. "The Logical Structure of Analytic Induction." *American Sociological Review* 16 (1951):812-18.

Rose, Arnold M., ed. *Human Behavior and Social Processes.* Boston: Houghton Mifflin, 1962.

————. "Interest in the Living Arrangements of the Urban Unattached." *American Journal of Sociology* 53 (1948):483-93.

————. "Living Arrangements of Unattached Persons." *American Sociological Review* 12 (1947):429-35.

Rose, Arnold M., and Peterson, Warren, eds. *Older People and Their Social World.* Philadelphia: F. A. Davis, 1965.

Rosenfelt, Rosalie M. "The Elderly Mystique." *Journal of Social Issues* 21 (1965):37-43.

Rosow, Irving. *Social Integration of the Aged.* Glencoe, Ill.: The Free Press, 1967.

Schwartz, Arthur, and Kleemeier, Robert. "The Effects of Illness and Age upon Some Aspects of Personality." *Journal of Gerontology* 20 (1965):85-91.

Shapiro, Joan H. "Dominant Leaders Among Slum Hotel Residents." *American Journal of Orthopsychiatry* 39 (1969):644-50.

————. "Reciprocal Dependence Between Single-room Occupancy Managers and Tenants." *Social Work* 15 (1970):67-73.

————. "Single-room Occupancy: Community of the Alone." *Social Work* 11 (1966):24-33.

Spradley, James P. *You Owe Yourself a Drunk: An Ethnography of Urban Nomads.* Boston: Little, Brown, 1970.

Stephens, Joyce. "The Aged Minority." *Occasional Papers in Gerontology* 10 (1971):59-63.

Streib, Gordon. "Morale of the Retired." *Social Problems* 3 (1956):270-76.

Tibbitts, Clark, and Donahue, Wilma, eds. *Social and Psychological Aspects of Aging.* New York: Columbia University Press, 1962.

Turner, Ralph H. "The Quest for Universals in Sociological Research." *American Sociological Review* 18 (1953):604-11.

Vidich, Arthur J., and Bensman, Joseph. "The Validity of Field Data." *Human Organization* 13 (1954):20-27.

Vidich, Arthur J., Bensman, Joseph, and Stein, Maurice R., eds. *Reflections on Community Studies.* New York: John Wiley and Sons, 1964.

Wax, Rosalie Hankey. "Twelve Years Later: An Analysis of Field Experience." *American Journal of Sociology* 63 (1957):133-42.

Webb, Eugene J. "Unconventionality, Triangulation, and Inference." *Proceedings of the 1966 International Conference on Testing Problems.* Princeton, N.J.: Educational Testing Service, 1966.

Webb, Eugene J., Campbell, Donald T., Schwartz, Richard D., and Sechrest, Lee. *Unobtrusive Measures: Nonreactive Research in the Social Sciences.* Chicago: Rand McNally, 1966.

Whyte, William Foote. *Street Corner Society.* Chicago: University of Chicago Press, 1943.

BIBLIOGRAPHY

Wilson, Thomas P. "Conceptions of Interaction and Forms of Sociological Explanation." *American Sociological Review* 35 (1970):697-710.

Wolverton, Charles. "Mysteries of the Carnival Language." *American Mercury* 35 (1935):227-31.

Wright, Richardson. *Hawkers and Walkers in Early America*. Philadelphia: J. B. Lippincott, 1927.

Znaniecki, Florian. *The Method of Sociology*. New York: Farrar and Rinehart, 1934.

Zorbaugh, Harvey Warren. *The Gold Coast and the Slum*. Chicago: University of Chicago Press, 1929.

―――. "The Dweller in Furnished Rooms: An Urban Type." In *The Urban Community*, edited by Ernest W. Burgess, pp. 98-105. Chicago: University of Chicago Press, 1926.